Technical Brief

Number 17

Imaging Techniques for Treatment Evaluation for Metastatic Breast Cancer

Prepared for:
Agency for Healthcare Research and Quality
U.S. Department of Health and Human Services
540 Gaither Road
Rockville, MD 20850
www.ahrq.gov

Contract No. 290-2012-00014-I

Prepared by:
Pacific Northwest Evidence-based Practice Center
University of Washington and
Oregon Health and Science University

Investigators:
Laura S. Gold, Ph.D.
Christoph I. Lee, M.D., M.S.H.S.
Beth Devine, Pharm.D., Ph.D.
Heidi Nelson, M.D., M.P.H.
Roger Chou, M.D.
Scott Ramsey, M.D., Ph.D.
Sean D. Sullivan, Ph.D.

AHRQ Publication No. 14-EHC044-EF
October 2014

This report is based on research conducted by the Pacific Northwest Evidence-based Practice Center under contract to the Agency for Healthcare Research and Quality (AHRQ), Rockville, MD (Contract No. 290-2012-00014-I). The findings and conclusions in this document are those of the authors, who are responsible for its contents; the findings and conclusions do not necessarily represent the views of AHRQ. Therefore, no statement in this report should be construed as an official position of AHRQ or of the U.S. Department of Health and Human Services.

The information in this report is intended to help health care decisionmakers—patients and clinicians, health system leaders, and policymakers, among others—make well informed decisions and thereby improve the quality of health care services. This report is not intended to be a substitute for the application of clinical judgment. Anyone who makes decisions concerning the provision of clinical care should consider this report in the same way as any medical reference and in conjunction with all other pertinent information, i.e., in the context of available resources and circumstances presented by individual patients.

This report may be used, in whole or in part, as the basis for development of clinical practice guidelines and other quality enhancement tools, or as a basis for reimbursement and coverage policies. AHRQ or U.S. Department of Health and Human Services endorsement of such derivative products may not be stated or implied.

This document is in the public domain and may be used and reprinted without special permission. Citation of the source is appreciated.

Persons using assistive technology may not be able to fully access information in this report. For assistance contact EffectiveHealthCare@ahrq.hhs.gov.

Suggested citation: Gold LS, Lee CI, Devine B, Nelson H, Chou R, Ramsey S, Sullivan SD. Imaging Techniques for Treatment Evaluation for Metastatic Breast Cancer. Technical Brief No. 17. (Prepared by the Pacific Northwest Evidence-based Practice Center under Contract No. 290-2012-00014-I.) AHRQ Publication No. 14-EHC044-EF. Rockville, MD: Agency for Healthcare Research and Quality; October 2014. www.effectivehealthcare.ahrq.gov/reports/final.cfm.

Preface

The Agency for Healthcare Research and Quality (AHRQ), through its Evidence-based Practice Centers (EPCs), sponsors the development of evidence reports and technology assessments to assist public- and private-sector organizations in their efforts to improve the quality of health care in the United States. The reports and assessments provide organizations with comprehensive, science-based information on common, costly medical conditions and new health care technologies and strategies. The EPCs systematically review the relevant scientific literature on topics assigned to them by AHRQ and conduct additional analyses when appropriate prior to developing their reports and assessments.

This EPC evidence report is a Technical Brief. A Technical Brief is a rapid report, typically on an emerging medical technology, strategy or intervention. It provides an overview of key issues related to the intervention—for example, current indications, relevant patient populations and subgroups of interest, outcomes measured, and contextual factors that may affect decisions regarding the intervention. Although Technical Briefs generally focus on interventions for which there are limited published data and too few completed protocol-driven studies to support definitive conclusions, the decision to request a Technical Brief is not solely based on the availability of clinical studies. The goals of the Technical Brief are to provide an early objective description of the state of the science, a potential framework for assessing the applications and implications of the intervention, a summary of ongoing research, and information on future research needs. In particular, through the Technical Brief, AHRQ hopes to gain insight on the appropriate conceptual framework and critical issues that will inform future comparative effectiveness research.

AHRQ expects that the EPC evidence reports and technology assessments will inform individual health plans, providers, and purchasers as well as the health care system as a whole by providing important information to help improve health care quality.

We welcome comments on this Technical Brief. They may be sent by mail to the Task Order Officer named below at: Agency for Healthcare Research and Quality, 540 Gaither Road, Rockville, MD 20850, or by email to epc@ahrq.hhs.gov.

Richard G. Kronick, Ph.D.
Director
Agency for Healthcare Research and Quality

Yen-pin Chiang, Ph.D.
Acting Deputy Director
Center for Evidence and Practice Improvement
Agency for Healthcare Research and Quality

Stephanie Chang, M.D., M.P.H.
Director
Evidence-based Practice Program
Center for Evidence and Practice Improvement
Agency for Healthcare Research and Quality

Elise Berliner, Ph.D.
Task Order Officer
Center for Evidence and Practice Improvement
Agency for Healthcare Research and Quality

Acknowledgments

The authors gratefully acknowledge the following individuals for their contributions to this project: Paul Kraegel, Elaine Graham, Andrew Hamilton, and Leah Williams.

Key Informants

In designing the study questions, the EPC consulted a panel of Key Informants who represent subject experts and end-users of research. Key Informant input can inform key issues related to the topic of the technical brief. Key Informants are not involved in the analysis of the evidence or the writing of the report. Therefore, in the end, study questions, design, methodological approaches and/or conclusions do not necessarily represent the views of individual Key Informants or their organizations.

Key Informants must disclose any financial conflicts of interest greater than $10,000 and any other relevant business or professional conflicts of interest. Because of their role as end-users, individuals with potential conflicts may be retained. The TOO and the EPC work to balance, manage, or mitigate any conflicts of interest.

The list of Key Informants who participated in developing this report follows:

Richard Frank, M.D., Ph.D.
Siemens Medical Solutions
Malvern, PA

John Hennessy
Sarah Cannon
Kansas City, MO

Jeff Hersh, Ph.D., M.D.
GE Healthcare
Wauwatosa, WI

Janie Lee, M.D., M.Sc.
University of Washington
Seattle, WA

Constance Lehman, M.D., Ph.D.
University of Washington
Seattle, WA

Gary Lyman, M.D., M.P.H.
Fred Hutchinson Cancer and Research
Center
Seattle, WA

David Mankoff, M.D., Ph.D.
University of Pennsylvania
Philadelphia, PA

Joanne Mortimer, M.D.
City of Hope
Duarte, CA

Mary Lou Smith, J.D., M.B.A.
Research Advocacy Network
Chicago, IL

Peer Reviewers

Prior to publication of the final evidence report, EPCs sought input from independent Peer reviewers without financial conflicts of interest. However, the conclusions and synthesis of the scientific literature presented in this report does not necessarily represent the views of individual reviewers.

Peer Reviewers must disclose any financial conflicts of interest greater than $10,000 and any other relevant business or professional conflicts of interest. Because of their unique clinical or content expertise, individuals with potential nonfinancial conflicts may be retained. The TOO and the EPC work to balance, manage, or mitigate any potential nonfinancial conflicts of interest identified.

The list of Peer Reviewers follows:

Leah Hole-Marshall, J.D.
Washington State Department of Labor and Industries
Olympia, WA

Hannah Linden, M.D.
University of Washington
Seattle, WA

Josh Morse, M.P.H.
Washington State Health Care Authority
Olympia, WA

Nina Mortazavi-Jehanno
Hôpital Rene Huguenin
Saint-Cloud, France

Robert Nordstrom, Ph.D.
National Cancer Institute
Bethesda, MD

Habib Rahbar, M.D.
University of Washington
Seattle, WA

Imaging Techniques for Treatment Evaluation for Metastatic Breast Cancer

Structured Abstract

Background. Although multiple imaging modalities to evaluate treatment response in patients with metastatic breast cancer are used clinically, their comparative effectiveness has not been determined.

Purpose. The purpose of this technical brief is to understand current utilization of metastatic breast imaging modalities for treatment evaluation in the United States, both in order to summarize the current state of the science and to inform future research on this topic.

Methods. We worked with Key Informants, including clinicians, patient advocates, representatives from the device manufacturing industry, and a product purchaser. Additionally, we searched gray and published literature from 2003 to 2013. We qualitatively synthesized the information from the Key Informant interviews and the gray literature. From the published literature, we abstracted data on the types of imaging used to evaluate treatment of metastatic breast cancer.

Findings. We identified bone scan (scintigraphy), magnetic resonance imaging (MRI), computed tomography (CT), and fluorodeoxyglucose-positron emission tomography (FDG-PET)/CT as the major modalities used for treatment evaluation of metastatic breast cancer in the United States. We also identified four types of imaging not commonly used currently that might become important within the next decade: F-fluoromisonidazole-(F-FMISO) PET/CT, fluorothymidine-(FLT) PET/CT, fluoroestradiol-(FES) PET/CT, and PET/MRI. All published reports pertaining to imaging evaluation of treatment response among metastatic breast cancer patients were limited to small observational studies. A review of the published literature found that, in general, uptake of tracers such as FDG in PET/CT scans is associated with tumor response as determined by bone scans, MRI, or CT.

Conclusions. Literature pertaining to imaging evaluation of treatment response among metastatic breast cancer patients was limited. An important potential advantage of FDG-PET/CT over conventional imaging for assessing tumor response among metastatic breast cancer patients is that it provides functional information regarding tumor metabolism in addition to information on gross morphologic changes. While some early evidence suggests that the metabolic response assessed by FDG-PET/CT after initial cycles of chemotherapy may be predictive of response to treatment among metastatic breast cancer patients, more rigorous research is needed before definitive conclusions can be reached. Future research efforts should focus on identifying novel radiotracers and biomarkers that may clarify breast tumor biology, addressing the lack of information on patient-centered outcomes (e.g., patient preferences) related to imaging, better delineating clinical outcomes associated with treatment response identified by imaging (e.g., progression-free and overall survival), and determining the costs associated with frequent imaging for treatment response.

Contents

Appendixes

Background

Introduction

In spite of significant gains in detection and treatment, breast cancer continues to have a broad impact in the United States, with an estimated 234,580 individuals with new diagnoses in 2013.[1] About 33 percent of individuals with breast cancer diagnosed between 2001 and 2007 had regional metastases, with a 5-year relative survival rate of 84 percent. Approximately 5 percent were diagnosed with distant metastases, most commonly to the bones, lungs, liver, or brain, and had a 5-year relative survival rate of only 23 percent.[1]

Several imaging modalities, including magnetic resonance imaging (MRI), computed tomography (CT), positron emission tomography (PET), PET/CT, and bone scintigraphy, are used to evaluate the effects of treatment for metastatic breast cancer.[2] However, as outlined in guidelines from the National Comprehensive Cancer Network and the National Institute for Health and Clinical Excellence, evidence regarding the accuracy and effectiveness of these modalities to evaluate treatment of metastatic breast cancer is lacking, even though the types and results of imaging may strongly affect patient outcomes.[2,3] Inappropriate use could lead to overtreatment. For example, use of CT during treatment response monitoring may show morphologic or size changes in the tumor in the setting of nonresponse, leading to continued ineffective and potentially toxic chemotherapy. Alternatively, inappropriate use of imaging may lead to undertreatment if foci of enlarging metastatic disease are not identified on CT and these lead to disease progression. Furthermore, imaging modalities vary substantially in cost, ranging in direct costs from about $250 for a bone scan to $1,114 for PET/CT,[4,5] underscoring the need to understand whether more expensive tests result in improved patient outcomes.

Current Practices in Imaging Metastatic Breast Cancer

In general, following diagnosis of metastatic breast cancer and initiation of treatment, women receive imaging about every 2–4 months in order to determine whether their tumor burden is improving. Since there are no reliable biomarkers to help determine response to treatment, oncologists are currently reliant mostly on visual detection of gross changes seen on imaging to guide treatment decisions. If imaging reveals that their cancer is progressing or is unchanged, alternative treatment regimens may be pursued. Although metastatic breast cancer is not curable, the goal of treatment is to prolong survival and reduce symptoms in order to maximize quality of life. Health care providers generally rely on recommendations from professional societies such as the National Comprehensive Cancer Network, the American Society for Clinical Oncology, and the European Society for Medical Oncology to guide the use of imaging techniques to assess treatment response in metastatic breast cancer. However, these recommendations are generally based on data that are not specific to assessing treatment in the metastatic breast cancer population. Current practice recommendations for managing metastatic breast cancer include imaging of the chest, abdomen, and bone in addition to obtaining medical histories, physical examinations, and relevant laboratory tests.[6,7] The most commonly used imaging modalities for treatment evaluation of metastatic breast cancer are chest/abdomen/pelvis CT and PET/CT.[6,7] For patients with bone-only metastases, bone scans are the most common imaging modality, with supplemental use of CT, MRI, and/or PET/CT to evaluate localized symptoms.[7,8]

Objective of This Technical Brief

Although multiple imaging modalities for treatment evaluation for metastatic breast cancer are used clinically, their comparative effectiveness in terms of health outcomes, patient satisfaction, and cost, has not been determined. The purpose of this technical brief is to understand current imaging utilization, emerging technologies, research in progress, patient values, and study design issues, in order to summarize the current state of the science and inform future research in this area. We evaluated whether imaging technologies were utilized differently among subpopulations and whether outcomes varied by subpopulations. We also evaluated the potential role of novel biomarkers in imaging for treatment evaluation of metastatic breast cancer. We combined information we obtained from published literature, gray literature, and Key Informants in order to provide the context for appropriate comparative effectiveness studies on imaging for treatment evaluation for metastatic breast cancer in the near future.

Guiding Questions

The questions below guided the data collection for this technical brief. Question 1 lays the groundwork for the literature review by describing each of the imaging modalities currently in use for treatment evaluation for metastatic breast cancer. We describe the accuracy, potential benefits, and potential risks of each modality, including safety, costs, adverse effects, and other issues. Question 2 provides the context for how each of the imaging modalities is currently used, including U.S. Food and Drug Administration (FDA) approval status, need for additional equipment (e.g., contrast agents), and, when possible, we describe reimbursement policies and how commonly each modality is used for metastatic breast cancer treatment evaluation. Using published studies and gray literature, Question 3 explores the state of the current research on the use and safety of each imaging modality. Finally, in Question 4, we identify important issues pertaining to metastatic breast cancer imaging, particularly areas of uncertainty surrounding ethical, economic, and safety issues, as well as areas of research that we expect to be pursued in the near future.

Guiding Question 1. Overview of Imaging Modalities Currently Used To Evaluate Treatment of Metastatic Breast Cancer

- What are the imaging modalities currently used for metastatic breast cancer treatment evaluation in the United States?
- What are the advantages, disadvantages, safety issues and relative costs of each modality?

Guiding Question 2. Context in Which Imaging Modalities Are Currently Used To Evaluate Treatment of Metastatic Breast Cancer

- What modalities have received FDA approval?
- What other resources (e.g., contrast agents, tracers) are commonly used with each modality?
- How commonly is each modality used?

Guiding Question 3. Current Evidence for Each Imaging Modality

- What published and unpublished studies have reported on the use and safety of each modality?

Guiding Question 4. Important Issues and Future Directions of Metastatic Breast Cancer Imaging for Treatment Evaluation

- Given the current state of the science, what are the implications for future diffusion of the imaging modalities for treatment evaluation of metastatic breast cancer?
- What are the economic, ethical, and privacy considerations that impact the diffusion of each imaging modality?
- What are important areas of uncertainty for metastatic breast cancer imaging modalities?
- What research questions would have the greatest individual and societal impact (e.g., in terms of how imaging for treatment evaluation affects survival time, quality of life, and health care utilization) for the population of women with metastatic breast cancer?

Methods

Overview

This technical brief combined systemic literature review approaches with Internet searches and Key Informant structured interviews and discussions.

Search Strategy

We first used broad search terms including Medical Subject Heading terms and key words related to imaging, metastatic breast cancer, and treatment evaluation. We conducted focused searches of PubMed® and the Cochrane Library. An experienced research librarian assisted us in choosing the search terms and limits (Appendix A). We also reviewed the reference lists of identified publications and added previously unidentified papers.

From these identified articles, we excluded publications that were beyond the scope of the technical brief (letters, comments, editorials, news, nonhuman studies, and articles not in English). Because imaging technologies are rapidly evolving, we excluded studies published prior to 2003. Searches were also conducted in a number of imaging and oncologic websites, including the American Society for Clinical Oncology, the American College of Radiology, the American Cancer Society, the National Comprehensive Cancer Network, and the Society for Nuclear Medicine. We also searched ClinicalTrials.gov, NIH Reporter, and ProQuest Dissertations and Theses to find unpublished studies. As in the published literature search, we excluded gray literature sources that were published prior to 2003, those that pertained to animal studies, and those that were not in English.

Eligibility Criteria

The inclusion and exclusion criteria are presented in Table 1. All titles and abstracts identified through searches were reviewed against our inclusion/exclusion criteria. For studies without adequate information to make a determination, we retrieved full-text articles and reviewed them against the inclusion/exclusion criteria.

Two team members (LG and CL) abstracted data from the published studies to provide an overview of the state of the science by collecting the following information:

- Study setting and geographic location
- Research design and methods
- Type(s) of imaging
- Breast cancer inclusion criteria
- Tumor factors (e.g., whether metastatic tumors were initially diagnosed or were recurrences)
- Comparators used
- Length of followup
- Outcomes associated with imaging findings (accurate detection of tumor response, changes in treatment decisions, prediction for survival, resource utilization, and adverse events).

We limited our data abstraction to studies dealing with imaging used to evaluate treatment response, and therefore did not identify any studies where imaging was an add-on or replacement for some other diagnostic tool aimed at treatment evaluation, or any studies where imaging was used for triaging patients for a future diagnostic test. Furthermore, we excluded studies that examined imaging that was used to detect recurrence after treatment had ended.

Table 1. Inclusion and exclusion criteria for imaging of metastatic breast cancer published literature search

Criterion	Inclusion	Exclusion
Population	Age 19 and above Females Diagnosed with metastatic (stage IV) breast cancer (initial diagnosis or recurrence)	Age 18 and below Males Diagnosed with stages I–III breast cancer Nonhuman
Indication for imaging	Imaging for treatment evaluation	Diagnostic imaging Imaging used to assess stage Imaging used to detect recurrence following successful treatment
Comparator	Comparison of multiple imaging modalities Tumor biomarkers No comparator	None
Outcomes associated with imaging findings	Tumor response Changes in treatment decisions Changes in patient decisions Recurrence-free survival Overall survival Quality of life Cost and resource utilization Adverse events	None
Timing	Published 2003–2013	Published 2002 or earlier
Setting	All care settings	None
Study design	Systematic reviews Randomized control trials Nonrandomized control trials Cohort studies (prospective and retrospective) Case-control studies Case series	Case reports Opinions Commentaries Letters to the editor with no primary data
Other	English language	Non-English language

Key Informant Discussions

We worked with the Key Informants to understand current imaging utilization practices, emerging technologies, research in progress, patient values, and study design issues, in order to help summarize the current state of the science and inform future research on imaging for treatment evaluation for women with metastatic breast cancer. We identified Key Informants including clinical experts/practitioners in radiology and oncology, as well as representatives of the patient perspective, product purchaser, and the device industry. Despite multiple attempts to identify a Key Informant to provide the perspective of health care entities that finance or reimburse for health costs, we could not identify one who was willing to serve in this capacity. Key Informants were identified through informal consultations with local, national, and international experts in breast cancer and imaging technologies. While we attempted to schedule more than one Key Informant per teleconference, most (n=5) calls consisted of only one Key Informant. Calls were led by one of several team members and at least two other team members participated. All calls were recorded for reference.

Initially, we asked the Key Informants to create a comprehensive list of imaging technologies, including technologies that are not commonly used or in development and may be used in the United States in the near future. We also asked them to identify the advantages and disadvantages and appropriateness of utilization of each type of imaging. Key Informants were asked to identify factors surrounding imaging decisions, including clinical guidelines, reimbursement policies, setting (e.g., tertiary care vs. community hospital), and patient preferences. The Key Informants also provided information about factors that patients consider when discussing imaging decisions with their providers such as test accuracy and invasiveness, safety issues, and out-of-pocket costs.

Findings

Overview

The availability of quantitative or qualitative data to address the guiding questions from our Key Informant interviews and the published and gray literature searches is presented in Table 2. Four imaging modalities are currently used in the United States for evaluating treatment response for metastatic breast cancer: bone scan, MRI, CT, and fluorodeoxyglucose (FDG)-PET/CT. We also identified four types of imaging not commonly used currently that might become important in the next 5–10 years: fluorothymidine (FLT)-PET/CT, F-fluoromisonidazole (F-FMISO)-PET/CT, fluoroestradiol (FES)-PET/CT, and PET/MRI.

In total, we interviewed nine Key Informants: five were clinicians (two of whom were medical oncologists who practiced at large academic institutions, two were radiologists at large academic institutions and one was a medical oncologist at a nonacademic research and treatment center), two were from product industry development companies, one was a patient advocate at a nonprofit advocacy organization, and one was an executive at a large cancer treatment center who provided both product purchaser and patient advocate perspectives. Three clinicians and one patient advocate were interviewed in the same phone call; all remaining calls were with only one Key Informant. Interviews lasted between 40–60 minutes and consisted of 8–13 questions. All interviews took place in October and November 2013. A summary of the interviews appears in Appendix B.

A summary of the findings from the published literature search is shown in Table 3 and the abstracted data are shown in Table 4. A full list of included and excluded studies is shown in Appendixes C and D. We abstracted data from a total of 17 publications.[9-25] Where the two abstractors disagreed, a discussion was performed to come to conclusions. The study populations from eight publications were from the United States,[9,14,19,20,22-25] eight were from Europe,[10,12,13,15-18,21] and one was from Asia.[11] All were cohort studies, of which seven were retrospective[10,14,17,19,20,23,24] and ten were prospective.[11-13,15,16,18,21,22,25] Twelve of seventeen studies[10-18,20,22,25] presented comparators pertaining to the type of imaging used; seven of these[10,13,15,16,18,20,22] compared metabolic response as measured by tracer uptake to response measured by anatomic imaging. Four studies[12,14,17,22] compared metabolic response measured by tracer uptake to measures of tumor biomarkers. One study[11] compared metabolic response as measured by two types of tracers (FDG- vs. F-FMISO-PET/CT). One study compared tumor response as assessed by bone scan compared with CT.[25] Almost all of the studies (16 of 17)[9-13,15-25] reported accuracy in detecting tumor response as an outcome. Seven[9,10,14-16,21,25] reported overall survival and four[14,17,23,25] reported progression-free survival. No studies reported recurrence-free survival, changes in treatment decisions, changes in patient decisions, quality of life, cost and resource utilization, or adverse events related to imaging. Only two studies[20,25] distinguished metastatic breast cancers that were initially diagnosed from those that were recurrences from nonmetastatic breast cancers. In total, the published literature reported on the imaging experiences of 557 women with metastatic breast cancer in the United States, Asia, and Europe. We estimate that approximately 792,000 women in the United States received imaging scans for the purpose of evaluating treatment of metastatic breast cancer (see Appendix F for details on this calculation) between 2003-2013, and thus the number of women enrolled in clinical studies to evaluate the benefits and harms of imaging for this purpose represented less than 0.1 percent of the women exposed to these procedures.

Finally, a summary of the findings from the gray literature search are shown in Table 5. We identified three current or soon-to-be recruiting clinical trials pertaining to imaging for treatment evaluation for metastatic breast cancer.

Summary of Imaging Trends for Treatment Evaluation of Metastatic Breast Cancer

We did not identify any studies that addressed imaging utilization trends for treatment evaluation of metastatic breast cancer. However, the Key Informants generally agreed that the trend of imaging for evaluation of treatment of metastatic breast cancer was toward stable or increased utilization; none speculated that imaging for this purpose would decrease in the near future. Additionally, the Key Informants identified several factors that may potentially influence utilization. For instance, all of the clinician, product purchaser, and patient advocate Key Informants reported that, in their experience, most payers readily reimburse for CT, PET-CT, bone scans, and other imaging modalities that are appropriate to the regions of the body where the metastases are located. However, the Key Informants indicated that some payers advocate for programs such as the use of Radiology Benefit Managers (entities used by private payers to require prior authorization) or peer-to-peer consultations (case discussions between ordering providers and radiologists), which may discourage physicians from ordering advanced imaging exams. Whether these mechanisms lead to more appropriate utilization is unclear. Several Key Informants also indicated that use of PET-CT can be influenced by the purchase of the expensive machinery and once the investment in the technology has been made, the scans will be used for many other indications besides treatment evaluation of metastatic breast cancer. One Key Informant indicated that insurance status might be more of a factor in community settings, with noninsured or underinsured patients being steered toward less expensive imaging. However, another Key Informant thought that physicians in academic centers might feel greater pressure to use more complicated and expensive technologies for fear of reprisals if they failed to order tests.

Summary of Shared Decisionmaking Regarding Imaging for Treatment Evaluation of Metastatic Breast Cancer

We did not find any published literature regarding patient involvement in decisionmaking regarding imaging for treatment evaluation of metastatic breast cancer. However, our Key Informants provided some information on this topic. They indicated that imaging is usually not the focus of patient education, both in terms of conversations that patients have with their care providers and the research that patients conduct on their own. Additionally, since physicians who interpret images usually interact with the ordering physicians rather than the patients themselves, patients are often under-informed about imaging and usually are not aware that they can engage in shared decisionmaking with their physicians regarding treatment evaluation by imaging.

Our Key Informants indicated that many patients are accustomed to receiving PET/CT and would not agree with receiving imaging followup only by CT after receipt of a previous PET/CT. Our Key Informants also reported that physicians might prefer to order tests based on their own experiences and biases, rather than spend time debating the merits of alternative imaging strategies with their patients.

Interestingly, the clinicians reported that they sometimes advocated for imaging less often to reduce the stress that patients feel while waiting for imaging results. Both Key Informant patient advocates reported that patients receive intangible value from receiving results of imaging scans that show their cancer is improving and are willing to experience the stress and anxiety of waiting for imaging results in order to potentially receive good news about their prognoses. Both patient advocates also reported that breast cancer patients are generally not concerned about the potential harm that could result from imaging, such as exposure to radiation from CT, PET, and PET/CT scans, because their therapies already involve such exposures.

Modalities Currently in Use

The imaging modalities currently in use and their key features, theoretical advantages, and theoretical disadvantaged are outlined in Table 6 and are described in more detail here.

Bone Scan (Scintigraphy)

Bone scans are used to identify areas of damage to the bones throughout the body. A small amount of a radionuclide tracer is injected intravenously and the patient is then scanned 2–3 hours later with a gamma camera that detects radiation emitted by the radioactive material. Areas of increased tracer uptake may indicate the presence of bone metastases. Although we could not find published data on how commonly bone scans are used to evaluate treatment of metastatic breast cancer, our Key Informants reported that bone scans are almost always used to evaluate treatment in patients who have been diagnosed with bony metastases. The Key Informants also reported that, because bone scans are less expensive than PET/CT, they may be ordered when PET/CT is not covered by the patient's insurance. Bone scans received FDA approval through the Medical Device Amendments of 1976, which allowed devices being clinically used to receive FDA approval without undergoing premarket approval or 510(k) clearance. The most commonly used radiotracer for bone scans is technetium-99m.[26] Safety issues pertaining to bone scans include exposure to radiation from the injected radiotracer and, rarely, the potential for allergic reactions. The Key Informants indicated that most patients were not concerned with exposure to radiation from imaging because their treatments usually entailed much larger doses.

We found three published studies that described use of bone scans to evaluate treatment of metastatic breast cancer.[10,20,25] Two compared PET tracer uptake (one evaluated FDG and the other evaluated FES) to bone scans and other types of anatomic imaging to determine tumor response. Although these studies were small (both had n=47), both studies found that the uptake of PET tracers were better predictors of response than bone scans (median response times were 6 and 87 months).[10,20] The third study stratified patients as having progressive disease or nonprogressive disease according to CT and bone scans. These authors found that treatment response identified by CT at 6 months was associated with progression-free survival, but treatment response demonstrated on bone scans at 6 months was not, and neither type of imaging at 6 months was associated with overall survival.[25]

Although we did not find specific information about the future directions of bone scans, our Key Informants indicated that the technology was extremely useful and was not likely to be displaced by other technologies in instances of bone metastases. None of the Key Informants prioritized bone scans as a potential topic for future research studies.

Magnetic Resonance Imaging

MRI scanners utilize strong magnetic fields and radio waves to create images of the body part of interest. The magnetic field emitted by the scanner causes hydrogen atoms that are components of water molecules in the patient's body to line up in the direction of the magnetic field so almost all of them point either to the patient's head or to their feet. A few atoms out of every million, however, are unmatched and do not point toward the head or the feet. When the radio frequency pulse is emitted, the unmatched atoms spin the opposite way. At the same time, gradient magnets arranged inside the main magnet are turned on and off quickly, creating radiowave signals that are captured by receiver coils and are used to construct images composed of the body part being scanned. For breast MRI, gadolinium-based contrast agents are also used to assist with evaluation of breast tumors. These contrast agents alter the local magnetic field of the breast tissue and allow visualization of abnormalities in the tissue being scanned. MRI scanners, breast coils, and gadolinium-based contrast agents have all received FDA approval.[27]

One potential advantage of MRI in comparison with other types of imaging such as CT and PET/CT is that MRI does not involve exposure to radiation.[28] Another potential advantage our Key Informants reported was that MRI was useful to evaluate treatment for patients with brain metastases who had received a baseline MRI. A potential disadvantage of MRI use is that the test may be difficult for claustrophobic patients to tolerate. Additionally, like bone scans, patients can experience allergic reactions to the contrast agents used for MRIs, but these are rare and most reactions are mild.[29] We did not find any quantitative evidence describing how commonly MRI is used to evaluate treatment of metastatic breast cancer.

We identified four published studies[9,15,16,20] that described use of MRI to evaluate treatment of metastatic breast cancer. Three of these compared treatment evaluation using tracer (FDG[15,16] and FES[20]) uptake from PET/CT with imaging using MRI and CT and one did not compare MRI to another method of treatment evaluation.[9] All three studies that compared conventional imaging and tracer uptake found correlations between tumor response using MRI and/or CT and PET radiotracer uptake.[15,16,20] However, only one of these reported data on the correlation between anatomic tumor response determined by MRI or CT and overall survival and found no correlation (mean followup time 27 weeks).[16]

Computed Tomography

CT uses a series of x-ray images taken around a rotating arc to reconstruct and generate three-dimensional images of structures in the body. The data from CT scanners are transmitted to computers, which create three-dimensional cross-sectional pictures. While CT scans are valuable in identifying and anatomically localizing tumors, they have disadvantages such as exposure to ionizing radiation and the potential for adverse events from iodinated contrast agents, which range from mild (nausea, itching) to severe (cardiopulmonary arrest).[30] Because CT systems were widely used prior to 1976, they received FDA approval through the Medical Device Amendments.[27]

Although we did not find published data on how commonly CT is used to monitor treatment of metastatic breast cancer, the clinical Key Informants reported that it is often used, especially in cases when staging PET/CT is not covered by insurance.

We identified seven published studies describing use of CT to evaluate treatment of metastatic breast cancer.[10,13,15,16,18,20,25] Most of these (n=5)[10,13,15,16,18] were conducted in Europe and all compared tracer uptake (FLT,[13,18] FDG,[10,15,16] and FES[20]) from PET/CT to anatomic imaging (including CT). Five of these studies found that uptake of the tracers was associated with changes in tumor volume measured by CT.[13,15,16,18,20] As described in the MRI section, another study reported no significant correlation between treatment-related changes seen on conventional imaging using CT or MRI and survival (mean followup time 27 weeks).[16] As described in the bone scan section, one study found that treatment-related changes seen on CT at

6 months were associated with progression-free survival, but changes seen on bone scans at 6 months were not, and neither was associated with overall survival.[25]

Positron Emission Tomography/Computed Tomography

A PET scan uses nuclear medicine imaging to produce three-dimensional color images of functional processes in the body. A patient is injected with a radioactive tracer and placed on a table that moves through a gamma ray detector array that contains a series of scintillation crystals. The crystals convert the gamma rays that are emitted from the patient into photons of light, which are amplified to electrical signals that are processed by a computer to generate images. The table is moved and the images are repeated so that a series of thin slice images of the body over the region of interest are assembled into a three-dimensional representation of the body. PET/CT scanners allow for a diagnostic CT scan to follow, providing anatomic correlation for the PET scan.

Several types of tracers have been developed for use with PET, including FDG, F-FMISO, FLT, and FES. FDG is the only tracer approved by the FDA for breast cancer imaging and is therefore the most widely used. Because tumors have increased glucose metabolism compared with noncancerous tissue, FDG has the ability to detect tumors on PET imaging. Specifically, tumor masses are relatively hypoxic compared with surrounding tissue, which activates the anaerobic glycolytic pathway. A consequence of enhanced glycolysis is the hyperactive trapping of FDG by tumor cells. Since 2006, all PET scanners purchased in the United States were combined PET/CT machines.[31] Like bone scans and computed tomography, PET scanners received FDA approval through the 1976 Medical Devices Amendment and combination PET/CT devices received 510(k) clearance in 2000.[27]

Our Key Informants indicated that FDG-PET/CT is currently the most commonly used type of imaging for treatment evaluation of metastatic breast cancer. The main potential advantage of PET/CT is its ability to combine the functional information from FDG uptake with the higher resolution of CT for determining anatomic location and tumor morphology. Both the PET and CT scans are obtained during the same exam and images are post-processed into a fused series of images. However, the modality does have potential disadvantages, including the relatively high cost of the test and exposure of the patients to ionizing radiation.[32] Largely because of these limitations, our Key Informants reported that they order PET/CT scans no more often than every 2-4 months during treatment for metastatic breast cancer, and only when patients are not obviously responding or worsening clinically.

Our Key Informants noted that PET/CT technology is relatively novel and few studies have prospectively evaluated long-term outcomes of its use in treatment evaluation for metastatic breast cancer. Additionally, the Key Informants felt PET/CT might be underused in community care settings, where access to a PET/CT machine might entail long travel times for patients or ordering physicians might not be accustomed to utilizing the technology.

Although the American College of Radiology provides accreditation of centers that use PET devices, they do not require standard procedures for preparing patients prior to their scan or require minimum interpretive volumes in order to remain accredited (as they do for breast MRI). Furthermore, interpretation of PET/CT scans is not monitored by any accrediting organization and no agencies exist to enforce the implementation of guidelines, resulting in inter-reader variability. The Key Informants also reported that PET/CTs for breast cancer are used relatively less frequently compared with PET/CTs for other solid organ malignancies, such that even at major cancer centers in large cities, only about 10 percent of the PET/CTs are related to breast cancer. Thus, the experience of PET/CT interpreting physicians for treatment evaluation of metastatic breast cancer may be somewhat limited due to relatively low volumes.

We identified a total of 15 studies describing use of PET to evaluate treatment for breast cancer.[10-24] Ten of these described use of FDG,[10,11,14-17,20,21,23,24] four described FLT,[12,13,18,22] one described F-FMISO,[11] and two described FES[19,20] (two studies evaluated more than one kind of tracer). Four studies evaluating FDG-PET,[10,15,16,20] two studies evaluating FLT-PET,[13,18] and one study evaluating FES-PET[20] compared tracer uptake values to anatomic imaging with MRI, bone scans, and/or CT, and these are described above.

Four studies compared tracer uptake (two looked at FDG[14,17] and two examined FLT[12,22]) with tumor biomarkers as ways to evaluate response to therapy. One study of 102 metastatic breast cancer patients found circulating tumor cells (CTCs) were correlated with FDG uptake in 67 percent of patients and, in univariate analyses, both FDG uptake and CTCs were predictive of survival; however, in multivariate analysis, FDG uptake was no longer predictive of survival.[14] The other study, conducted in Belgium (n=25), found only 28 percent concordance between FDG uptake and the tumor markers CA15-3 or carcinoembryonic antigen. This study did find a longer progression-free survival in patients who showed response on FDG-PET (11 months) compared with patients who were nonresponders (7 months).[17] For the studies examining FLT, although sample sizes were small (n=14 and n=9), both found correlations between uptake of FLT and tumor markers (CA27.29 and CTCs).[12,22] Additionally, one of the studies reported strong correlations between a baseline FLT-PET scan and a repeat scan 2−10 (median 4.5) days later (r=0.99 for standardized uptake value at 90 minutes between the scans at the two time points).[18] This was the only study that we identified that presented results on the reproducibility of an imaging modality.

Three studies reported on disease progression by standard FDG uptake values.[21,23,24] All reported that standardized uptake values on initial FDG-PET scans were associated with outcomes, including time to disease progression or skeletal-related event (n=28; median followup 17.5 months),[23] response duration (n= 102; median followup=15 months),[24] and progression-free survival (n=22; followup was at least 4 years).[21]

One small study[19] (n=30, 27 of which were women) reported use of FES-PET to compare response to estrogen blocking therapy with estrogen depleting therapy in patients with bone metastases undergoing salvage endocrine therapy. These authors found the standardized uptake value of FES declined 54 percent in patients taking estrogen-blocking therapy and declined only 14 percent for patients taking estrogen-depleting agents.[19] Finally, one small study[11] (n=12) conducted in China compared use of F-FMISO to FDG-PET. While FDG uptake did not correlate with clinical outcomes, F-FMISO-PET showed a fairly strong correlation (r=0.77).[11]

Positron Emission Tomography/Magnetic Resonance Imaging

Several of our Key Informants mentioned that combination PET/MRI scanners might become important within the next decade and at least one such device has received FDA approval.[33] However, we did not find any published or gray literature describing use of this modality to evaluate treatment of metastatic breast cancer. Although a major disadvantage of this technology is that it combines two expensive modalities, it might be ideal for imaging of brain metastases. By combining PET's metabolic imaging capabilities with MRI's excellent tissue contrast, the combination may increase accuracy in evaluating response to therapy for brain metastases. Another advantage is that, unlike PET/CT, it would not involve exposure to as much ionizing radiation from the CT component (although it would still entail some radiation exposure from the tracer).[34]

Table 2. Availability of data in Key Informant interviews, published literature, and gray literature to address guiding questions

	Modalities Currently in Use: Bone Scan	Modalities Currently in Use: MRI	Modalities Currently in Use: CT	Modalities Currently in Use: FDG-PET/CT	Investigational: FLT-PET/CT	Investigational: F-FMISO-PET/CT	Investigational: FES-PET/CT	Investigational: PET/MRI
GQ 1: Overview of Imaging Modalities								
a. What modalities are currently being used in the United States?	KI, PL, GL	KI, PL, GL	KI, PL, GL	KI, PL, GL	KI, PL, GL	PL	KI, PL, GL	KI
b. Advantages and disadvantages of each?	KI, PL	KI, PL	KI, PL	KI, PL				
GQ 2: Context of Use								
a. FDA status	PL	PL	PL	PL	PL	PL	PL	PL
b. Contrast agents used	PL	PL	PL	PL	PL	PL	PL	
c. How commonly is modality used?	KI, PL	KI, PL	KI, PL	KI, PL	KI, PL	PL	KI, PL	KI, PL
GQ 3: Current Evidence								
a. Patient population	KI, PL	KI, PL	KI, PL	KI, PL	KI, PL	PL	KI, PL	
b. Study design/size	PL	PL	PL	PL	PL	PL	PL	
c. Concurrent/prior imaging				PL				
d. Length of followup	PL	PL	PL	PL	PL	PL	PL	
e. Outcomes	PL	PL	PL	PL	PL	PL	PL	
f. Adverse events			KI, PL	KI, PL	KI, PL	KI, PL	KI, PL	
GQ 4: Issues and Future Directions								
a. Future diffusion of the modality?				KI			KI	KI
b. Economic and ethical considerations?	KI			KI				KI
c. Final decisions about ordering?	KI			KI				
d. Areas of uncertainty/priority research questions?				KI	KI		KI	KI

CT = computed tomography; F-FMISO = F-fluoromisonidazole; FDA = U.S. Food and Drug Administration; FDG = fluorodeoxyglucose; FES = fluoroestradiol; FLT = fluorothymidine; GL = gray literature; GQ = guiding question; KI = Key Informant; MRI = magnetic resonance imaging; PET = positron emission tomography; PL = published literature

14

Table 3. Overview of published literature (n=17 studies[a]), with number of metastatic breast cancer patients (n=557)

	Bone Scan (n=3 studies; 123 patients)	MRI (n=4 studies; 130 patients)	CT (n=7 studies; 206 patients)	FDG-PET or FDG-PET/CT (n=10 studies; 454 patients)	FLT-PET/CT (n=4 studies; 33 patients)	F-FMISO PET/CT (n=1 study; 12 patients)	FES-PET/CT (n=2 studies; 74 patients)	Total (n=17 studies; 557 patients)
Study Population								
United States	2 (n=76)	2 (n=61)	2 (n=76)	4 (n=279)	1 (n=14)	0	2 (n=74)	8 (n=273)
Europe	1 (n=47)	2 (n=69)	5 (n=130)	5 (n=163)	3 (n=19)	0	0	8 (n=272)
Asia	0	0	0	1 (n=12)	0	1 (n=12)	0	1 (n=12)
Study Type								
Cohort (retrospective)	2 (n=94)	1 (n=47)	2 (n=94)	6 (n=351)	0	0	2 (n=74)	7 (n=378)
Cohort (prospective)	1 (n=29)	3 (n=83)	5 (n=112)	4 (n=103)	4 (n=33)	1 (n=12)	0	10 (n=179)
Randomized control trial	0	0	0	0	0	0	0	0
Comparators[b]								
Tracer uptake vs. anatomic imaging	2 (n=94)	3 (n=116)	6 (n=177)	4 (n=163)	3 (n=28)	0	1 (n=47)	7 (n=191)
2 tracer uptakes	0	0	0	1 (n=12)	0	1 (n=12)	0	1 (n=12)
Tracer uptake vs. biomarkers	0	0	0	2 (n=127)	2 (n=19)	0	0	4 (n=146)
Bone scan vs. anatomic imaging	1 (n=29)	0	1 (n=29)	0	0	0	0	1 (n=29)
Outcomes[c]								
Tumor response	3 (n=123)	3 (n=116)	7 (n=206)	10 (n=454)	4 (n=33)	1 (n=12)	2 (n=74)	16 (n=543)
Progression-free survival	1 (n=29)	0	1 (n=29)	3 (n=149)	0	0	0	4 (n=178)
Overall survival	1 (n=76)	3 (n=83)	4 (n=145)	5 (n=240)	0	0	0	5 (n=283)

CT = computed tomography; F-FMISO = F-fluoromisonidazole; FDG = fluorodeoxyglucose; FES = fluoroestradiol; FLT = fluorothymidine; MRI = magnetic resonance imaging; PET = positron emission tomography

[a] Eight studies included greater than one type of imaging

[b] Five studies did not include comparators of imaging

[c] Some studies reported greater than one outcome

Table 4. Abstracted data from published literature

Author Year	Study Design	Inclusion/Exclusion Criteria	N	Age (mean, range)	Imaging Modalities	Comparators	Tumor Response	Overall Survival	Timing Outcome Measures	Setting	Location
Buijs 2007[9]	Retrospective case series	MBC; receipt of MRI	14	57 (41-81)	MRI	None	NA	25 months	3 years	Single institution	United States
Cachin 2006[10]	Retrospective cohort	MBC; post-stem transplant PET scans	47	44 (26-60)	FDG-PET; CT, ultrasound, mammogram, bone scan	FDG-PET vs. conventional imaging	Conventional imaging: 37% complete response; FDG-PET, 72% achieved complete response.	19 months	87 month	Single institution	France
Cheng 2013[11]	Prospective cohort	Post-menopausal, ER+ BC, stages II-IV	12	65.1 (55-82)	FDG-PET/CT; F-FMISO-PET/CT	FDG-PET/CT vs. F-FMISO-PET/CT	FDG did not correlate with clinical outcomes; F-FMISO did correlate (r=0.77)	NR	3 month	Single institution	China
Contractor 2012[12]	Prospective cohort	MBC	5	NR	FLT-PET/CT	Change in FLT uptake vs. change in CTCs	FLT uptake correlated with decrease CTCs	NR	2 weeks	Single institution	United Kingdom
Contractor 2011[13]	Prospective cohort	Stage II-IV BC with lesion outside bone/liver	20 (9 with stage IV)	54 (41-69)	FLT-PET/CT	FLT-PET SUV vs. anatomic response from CT	Reduction SUV associated with lesion size changes	NR	3 cycles of treatment	Single institution	United Kingdom
De Giorgi 2009[14]	Retrospective cohort	MBC	102	55.5 (SD 10.8)	FDG-PET/CT	FDG SUV vs. CTCs	CTC levels correlated with FDG uptake	15.7 +/- 7.8 months	9-12 weeks	Single institution	United States
Dose Schwartz 2005[15]	Prospective cohort	MBC	11	49 (34-68)	FDG-PET	FDG-PET vs. conventional imaging	FDG uptake correlated with conventional imaging response	14.5 months	27 weeks	Single institution	Germany

Table 4. Abstracted data from published literature (continued)

Author Year	Study Design	Inclusion/Exclusion Criteria	N	Age (mean, range)	Imaging Modalities	Comparators	Tumor Response	Overall Survival	Timing Outcome Measures	Setting	Location
Haug 2012[16]	Prospective cohort	MBC to liver and life expectancy of >3 months	58	58 (SD 11)	FDG-PET/CT; CT, MRI of liver	FDG-PET vs. CT and MRI	NR	47 weeks	27 weeks	Single institution	Germany
Hayashi 2013[25]	Prospective cohort	MBC	29	53 (30-91)	CT, bone scan	Patients stratified into progressive/ non progressive disease by bone scan and CT	Progressive/ non progressive disease using CT or bone scan not predictive of progression free survival at 3 months; CT predictive at 6 months	Progressive/ non progressive disease using CT or bone scan not predictive of overall survival at 3 or 6 months	26.7 months	Single institution	United States
Huyge 2010[17]	Retrospective cohort	MBC to bone with 2 PET/CTs	25	52 (37-72)	FDG PET/CT	FDG-PET/CT vs. CA15-3 or CEA	28% concordance PET/CT and tumor markers	NR	3 months	Single institution	Belgium
Kenny 2007[18]	Prospective cohort	Stage II-IV BC; life expectancy >3 months	5 stage IV	54 (36-80)	FLT-PET/CT	FLT-PET/CT 1 week after therapy initiation to clinical response (as measured by PET) at 60 days	FLT response correlated with clinical response. FLT response preceded tumor size change	NR	60 days	Single institution	United Kingdom
Linden 2006[20]	Retrospective cohort	MBC, ER + cancer with > 6 months followup	47	56 (35-76)	FES-PET	FES-PET vs. clinical response	Correlation between FES SUV and clinical response	0 patients had complete response to endocrine therapy; 23% had partial response	6 months	Single institution	United States

17

Table 4. Abstracted data from published literature (continued)

Author Year	Study Design	Inclusion/ Exclusion Criteria	N	Age (mean, range)	Imaging Modalities	Comparators	Tumor Response	Overall Survival	Timing Outcome Measures	Setting	Location
Linden 2011[19]	Retrospective cohort	MBC to bone, salvage endocrine therapy	27	55 (28-77)	FES-PET	None	NR	NR	6 weeks	Single institution	United States
Mortazavi-Jehanno 2012[21]	Prospective cohort	MBC with endocrine therapy	22	58 (40-82)	FDG PET/CT	Progression free, overall survival by different levels of SUV max	NR	55 months partial response; 71 months stable disease; 52 months progressive disease group (NSD)	4 years	Single institution	France
Pio 2006[22]	Prospective cohort	MBC	14	NR	FLT-PET	Compared FLT uptake to CA27.29 tumor marker levels and tumor size by CT	FLT uptake good predictor of change in tumor size on CT; also correlated with change in CA27.29	NR	5.8 months	Single institution	United States
Specht 2007[23]	Retrospective cohort	MBC to bone with 2 PETs	28	51 (30-68)	FDG-PET	Time to progression by level of SUV max	Changes in FDG SUV associated with time to progression	NR	17.5 months; only 1 death	Single institution	United States
Tateishi 2008[24]	Retrospective Cohort	MBC to bone with PET/CT	102	55 (25-89)	FDG-PET/CT	Baseline vs. post-treatment tumor factors	SUV decrease predicted response duration	NR	15 months	Single institution	United States

BC = breast cancer; CA15-3 = cancer antigen 15-3; CA27-29 – cancer antigen 27-29; CEA = carcinoembryonic antigen; CT = computed tomography; CTCs = circulating tumor cells; ER+ = estrogen receptor positive; F-FMISO = F-fluoromisonidazole; FES = fluoroestradiol; FLT = fluorothymidine; MBC = metastatic breast cancer; MRI = magnetic resonance imaging; NA = not applicable; NR = not reported; NSD = no significant difference; PET = positron emission tomography; SD = standard deviation; SUV = standardized uptake value

18

Table 5. Overview of gray literature findings

Website	Identifier	Type(s) of Imaging	Study Design	Institution	Estimated Enrollment & Eligibility	Primary Outcome Measure(s)	Area(s) of imaging	Study Status Nov 2013
Clinicaltrials.gov	NCT01621906	MRI, FLT-PET	Prospective Cohort (nonrandomized)	Memorial Sloan-Kettering Cancer Center, New York, United States	N=20; histologically confirmed metastatic adenocarcinoma of breast with brain metastases with planned whole brain radiation therapy.	Tumor response measured anatomically with MRI compared with SUV from FLT-PET	Brain Metastases	Recruiting
Clinicaltrials.gov	NCT01805908	111 Indium-Pertuzumab SPECT-CT	Prospective Cohort (nonrandomized)	Ontario Clinical Oncology Group, Canada	N=30; metastatic adenocarcinoma of breast; tumor HER2 positive; initiating treatment with Trastuzumab.	Change in tumor SUV from baseline to day 8; toxicities attributable to 111 Indium Pertuzumab injections	Whole body	Not yet recruiting
Clinicaltrials.gov	NCT01627704	FES-PET	Prospective Cohort (nonrandomized)	Assistance Publique-Hopitaux de Paris, France	N=72; metastatic adenocarcinoma of breast with hormone-dependent cancer.	Tumor response according to FES SUV 6 months after induction or major change in hormone therapy	Whole body	Recruiting
NIH Reporter	5P01CA042045-24	FLT-PET; MRI; FES-PET	Not stated	University of Washington, Seattle, WA, United States	Not stated	Not stated	Whole body	Ongoing

CT = computed tomography; FES = fluoroestradiol; FLT = fluorothymidine; HER2 = Human Epidermal Growth Factor Receptor-2; MRI = magnetic resonance imaging; PET = positron emission tomography; SPECT = single-photon emission computed tomography; SUV = standardized uptake value

Table 6. Imaging modalities and key characteristics

Imaging Modality	Key Characteristics	Theoretical Advantage(s)	Theoretical Disadvantage(s)
Bone scan (scintigraphy)	- Detection of radiation emitted by injected radioactive tracer with use of a gamma camera to create two-dimensional images of the body	- Measures bone remodeling and turnover; can detect bone turnover of 5-15% from normal - Relatively inexpensive compared with other imaging modalities	- Cannot identify destructive (lytic) bone lesions well - Requires exposure to ionizing radiation - Poorer anatomic localization and tumor morphology compared with other imaging modalities
Magnetic resonance imaging	- Uses strong magnetic fields and radiowaves to create three-dimensional images of the body - Requires intravenous gadolinium contrast injection	- No exposure to ionizing radiation - Excellent anatomic localization of brain metastases (if baseline MRI obtained)	- No functional information regarding tumor metabolism - Relatively expensive compared with other imaging modalities - Difficult for claustrophobic patients to tolerate - Poorer anatomic localization than PET/CT for chest, abdomen, pelvis
Computed tomography (CT)	- Series of x-ray images reconstructed into three-dimensional images of the body - Requires intravenous iodinated contrast injection	- Excellent anatomic localization and tumor morphology visualization	- No functional information regarding tumor metabolism - Requires exposure to ionizing radiation - Adverse reactions to iodinated contrast material not uncommon
Positron-emission tomography/Computed tomography	- Scintillation crystals convert gamma rays into photons which are amplified to electronic signals used to create three-dimensional images - Requires intravenous injection of radioactive tracer - CT scan obtained during same exam and images fused with PET images	- Combines functional information from FDG uptake (glucose metabolism of tumors) with high resolution of CT for anatomic localization and tumor morphology visualization	- Relatively expensive compared with other imaging modalities - Requires exposure to ionizing radiation from both radioactive tracer and CT scan
Positron-emission tomography/Magnetic resonance imaging	- Scintillation crystals convert gamma rays into photons which are amplified to electronic signals used to create three-dimensional images - Requires intravenous injection of radioactive tracer and gadolinium contrast - MRI scan obtained during the same exam and images fused with PET images	- May be ideal for imaging of brain metastases - Less exposure to ionizing radiation compared with PET/CT	- Combines two relatively expensive imaging modalities - Difficult for claustrophobic patients to tolerate

CT = computed tomography; MRI = magnetic resonance imaging; PET = positron-emission tomography

Summary and Implications

Currently, there is a relatively small amount of published reports pertaining to imaging evaluation of treatment response among metastatic breast cancer patients. Most reports were from small, single-institution, nonrandomized observational studies. Our review of the literature, along with Key Informant opinion, suggested that FDG-PET/CT is the imaging modality of choice for assessing tumor response among metastatic breast cancer patients over conventional imaging (including CT, MRI, and bone scintigraphy). This preference is due to FDG-PET/CT theoretically providing information regarding functional tumor response to chemotherapy or hormone therapy by measuring changes in tumor metabolism, whereas conventional imaging can only demonstrate gross morphologic changes of tumors in a delayed fashion. Moreover, some early evidence suggested that the metabolic response assessed by FDG-PET/CT after initial cycles of chemotherapy may be predictive of response to treatment among metastatic breast cancer patients, but more rigorous research is needed before definitive conclusions can be reached.

Nevertheless, conventional imaging by CT, MRI, and bone scintigraphy are the most common comparators in studies evaluating the ability of FDG-PET/CT to determine tumor response and are also considered appropriate care. The choice of imaging modality for conventional imaging is dependent upon the location of known metastases (e.g., MRI is best for evaluating brain metastases, CT is best for evaluating lung metastases, and bone scintigraphy is best for evaluating skeletal metastases). The few studies evaluating specific sites of breast cancer metastases pertained to the bone, demonstrating improved response detection for PET/CT over conventional imaging. However, larger-scale studies are required to truly demonstrate the comparative effectiveness of PET/CT and conventional imaging for specific sites of breast cancer metastases with regard to outcomes such as progression-free survival, and decreased chemotoxicity, with earlier stoppage of ineffective therapies. In particular, we did not find reports in the published literature on changes in treatment decisions following the various types of imaging, which could provide information on whether changes identified by different modalities were more likely to alter treatment regimens and, in turn, affect survival times. Changes in treatment regimen may be a particularly important outcome to study in women with bone dominant metastatic breast cancer, since healing bones may appear as "flares" on bone scans, and treatment that is, in fact, working, may inappropriately be changed. Bone dominant metastatic patients have largely been excluded from published studies on treatment response by imaging, and represent an area in need of further research.

The major limitation noted by both the available studies and Key Informants regarding PET/CT for evaluating treatment response is the mechanism of FDG, the only FDA-approved radiotracer for breast cancer imaging. FDG is an indicator of glucose metabolism within cells rather than a direct measure of tumor proliferation. Small pilot studies have reported on the efficacy of several novel tracers that may be able to measure tumor behavior at the molecular level more directly. With a majority of breast cancer patients having estrogen-receptor positive disease, FES may be able to predict the response of metastatic breast cancers to hormonal therapy (e.g., tamoxifen) and to help guide treatment decisions. FLT is another novel radiotracer that was developed as a marker for cellular proliferation, and it may be less susceptible to early inflammatory response to therapy compared with FDG. Future research on novel radiotracers may help clarify heterogeneous breast cancer tumor biology and allow discovery of treatments that might be successful in improving outcomes.

Another major limitation of the published literature on imaging used for treatment evaluation of metastatic breast cancer was the lack of description of potential sources of noise and bias in the imaging machines and protocols that were described in the studies. Although many of the reviewed published literature studies examined small populations of metastatic breast cancer patients who received their scans on the same machines with the same imaging protocols, only one study[18] published data on the reproducibility of scans at different time points. This is especially an issue for women who receive imaging from different devices, or even imaging facilities, over the course of their cancer treatment. Future studies should provide information on the quantitative characteristics of the imaging devices so that comparative effectiveness results can be obtained.

Beyond using conventional imaging as a comparator to PET/CT, a few pilot studies have also attempted to evaluate the efficacy of measuring CTCs as biomarkers for therapeutic monitoring in metastatic breast cancer patients. Early data are inconclusive as to whether measuring CTCs has added value beyond functional PET/CT imaging for assessing immediate response to chemotherapy. With regard to new imaging modalities, PET/MRI may hold promise in the evaluation of metastases to the brain; however, it is not currently in wide use. Both biomarkers like CTCs and novel imaging modalities like PET/MRI warrant further development and evaluation in select subpopulations of metastatic breast cancer patients.

The most glaring knowledge gap with regard to imaging evaluation for treatment response in metastatic breast cancer was the evaluation of patient-centered outcomes. None of the published studies examined how the imaging experience or imaging findings affected patient satisfaction, patient anxiety levels, or other outcome measures that may be of central importance to metastatic breast cancer patients beyond survival benefit. Based on Key Informant input, metastatic breast cancer patients are currently under-informed regarding the role of medical imaging in determining treatment response and its ability to guide treatment decisions. Patients are also under-informed with regard to the alternatives to monitoring response by imaging. Future research efforts should address patient-centered outcome measures and shared decision-making associated with imaging evaluation for treatment response.

Finally, no studies addressed the issue of resource use and costs associated with imaging evaluation for treatment response for metastatic breast cancer. However, if PET/CT can correctly predict response as early as the first cycle of chemotherapy, then the relatively high cost associated with the modality may be outweighed by the potential cost savings from avoiding multiple additional cycles of ineffective chemotherapy and associated potential chemotoxicity. Out-of-pocket costs associated with imaging evaluation were also a concern among patients according to our Key Informants. The associated direct and indirect costs of PET/CT compared with conventional imaging should be examined in parallel with outcomes of future studies in order to determine the true value of different imaging modalities for evaluating treatment response among metastatic breast cancer patients.

Next Steps

Key Informants identified future research needs in several areas that they thought would have large impacts on clinical decisionmaking regarding imaging for treatment evaluation of metastatic breast cancer. Ideally, a treatment evaluation tool would, within days or weeks of beginning treatment, be able to accurately and noninvasively detect whether the treatment was reducing cancer burden without exposing women to potentially harmful side effects such as contrast reactions or ionizing radiation. Such a tool (e.g., a blood test) would ideally be inexpensive, readily accessible to women with metastatic breast cancer, and potentially replace the need for imaging evaluation for treatment response.

Intermediate and Long-Term Outcomes

Several Key Informants were interested in research that examines clinical and patient-centered outcomes to determine the impact that choice of imaging technologies has on survival, treatment selection, cost, and quality of life. Key Informants were also interested in examining how often more advanced imaging (e.g., PET/CT scans) should be conducted to evaluate treatment in order to lead to the best intermediate and long-term outcomes. Additionally, we did not find any evidence in the published literature about the extent of imaging that is ideal during treatment. For example, if only one site of metastasis is found in initial imaging, should future imaging for treatment evaluation include other potential sites of metastasis to document treatment failure and further spread of disease? Because metastatic breast cancer cannot be cured, the ultimate goal of treatment is to prolong survival with the least reduction in quality of life. Ideally, research into intermediate and long-term outcomes would identify imaging that indicates when treatments are not working as soon as possible so treatment can be stopped, potentially toxic side effects can be minimized, and other forms of treatment can be pursued.

One potential research design that could answer such questions would be to randomize women with metastatic breast cancer to different imaging regimens prior to beginning treatment with followup imaging using the same modalities and imaging protocols at varying time intervals to assess how the modality and timing of imaging affects outcomes. To minimize confounding, randomization could be multi-pronged to account for important clinical differences. For example, randomization could be done separately depending on estrogen receptor status since women with estrogen receptor-positive disease typically have longer survival times and may benefit from different imaging regimens compared with women with estrogen receptor-negative disease. Women would be followed until death or 3 years after diagnosis and cancer recurrences and treatment selections could be assessed from electronic medical records. Additionally, all costs incurred during the followup period could be compared between the different imaging arms. Women could also be surveyed at 6-month intervals to assess quality of life. The time and cost that would be necessary to conduct such a study would be substantial and confounding factors, such as patient and physician imaging and treatment preferences, might make a traditional, multi-institution randomized trial methodologically difficult.

Alternative approaches to examining intermediate and long-term patient-centered outcomes include the use of more adaptive trial designs, such as a pragmatic trial design that allows greater freedom regarding patient and physician imaging and treatment decisions. Even a prospective observational study design involving multiple institutions would provide valuable information regarding the effects of imaging modalities and the frequency of imaging on outcomes. A quality-of-life survey instrument can be easily implemented in either the pragmatic trial or prospective observational study designs to capture patient perspectives on treatment evaluation by imaging. Finally, decision analysis and simulation modeling may have a critical role in estimating the effects of imaging modality and frequency on the intermediate and long-term outcomes for metastatic patients given the time and cost barriers for performing traditional randomized trials.

Improving Communication With Patients

Studies that focus on improving communication with patients regarding imaging for the purpose of assessing treatment for metastatic breast cancer would be of interest. One option to begin to explore this topic would be to convene focus groups of women who are currently undergoing or have recently completed treatment for metastatic breast cancer and ask targeted questions about their patient-physician communication experiences about imaging. These groups could help researchers gain understanding about the particular research questions that are important to this patient population and would identify the key patient-centered outcomes that should be studied through the aforementioned potential study designs.

For instance, Key Informants were relatively less concerned about ionizing radiation exposure from advanced imaging than initially expected. It is uncertain whether this sentiment is more widespread, or if there remain a large number of patients and providers who are concerned about potential radiation risks. An area of improved communication with patients and providers, therefore, would be to increase stakeholder awareness of the innovative, dose-lowering technologies that have been implemented over the last several years to minimize potential harm from radiation associated with CT, PET, and bone scans. These technologies include automatic exposure control and iterative reconstruction of CT images, as well as advanced electronics in imaging data acquisition systems that limit exposure time. Overall, greater communication between providers and patients may be required to clarify the balance between the benefits and harms of imaging during the informed consent process.

Personalized Medicine

Key Informants were also interested in imaging that could characterize tumors at the genetic or proteomic level and allow treatments to be specific to particular types of breast cancer, given that breast cancer is a heterogenous disease. Truly personalized imaging for treatment response would require further development of new radiotracers specific to the biological nature of individual breast cancers. More rigorous evaluation of novel radiotracers such as FES and FLT are needed to determine their comparative effectiveness to standard FDG use with PET/CT in specific patient subpopulations.

Blood Tests To Evaluate Treatment

Several Key Informants indicated that research on biomarkers that could evaluate treatment response and obviate the need for imaging would be greatly useful. There is currently insufficient evidence regarding CTCs and whether their measurement can help predict survival time for metastatic breast cancer patients. There is also insufficient evidence regarding whether measuring such blood tumor markers can guide treatment choices for metastatic breast cancer better than current use of advanced imaging modalities. Future research efforts should focus on the comparative predictive power of CTCs for treatment response and survival versus PET/CT and/or anatomic imaging for treatment response.

References

1. American Cancer Society. Cancer Facts & Figures 2013. Atlanta, GA: 2013. www.cancer.org/acs/groups/content/@epide miologysurveilance/documents/document/ac spc-036845.pdf. Accessed November 6, 2013.

2. National Comprehensive Cancer Network Inc. Breast Cancer. NCCN; 3/11/2013 2013. www.nccn.org/professionals/physician_gls/p df/breast.pdf. Accessed November 6, 2013

3. National Institute for Health and Clinical Excellence (NICE). Advanced Breast Cancer: Diagnosis and Treatment National Collaborating Centre for Cancer National Institute for Health and Clinical Excellence. London: 2009. www.nice.org.uk/nicemedia/live/11778/433 05/43305.pdf. Accessed November 6, 2013.

4. Centers for Medicare and Medicaid Services (CMS). Physician Fee Schedule. 2009. http://chfs.ky.gov/nr/rdonlyres/4fd6f67c-6c97-4061-a9fd-2441467201f2/0/mdfee2009rev4909r2.pdf. Accessed November 6, 2013.

5. Centers for Medicare and Medicaid Services (CMS). Medicare Program: Changes to the Hospital Outpatient Prospective Payment System and CY 2009 Payment Rates CMS. 2009. www.cms.gov/Medicare/Medicare-Fee-for-Service-Payment/HospitalOutpatientPPS/downloads/ CMS-1404-FC.pdf

6. Cardoso F, Costa A, Norton L, et al. 1st International consensus guidelines for advanced breast cancer (ABC 1). Breast. 2012 Jun;21(3):242-52. PMID: 22425534.

7. Lin NU, Thomssen C, Cardoso F, et al. International guidelines for management of metastatic breast cancer (MBC) from the European School of Oncology (ESO)-MBC Task Force: Surveillance, staging, and evaluation of patients with early-stage and metastatic breast cancer. Breast. 2013 Jun;22(3):203-10. PMID: 23601761.

8. Costelloe CM, Rohren EM, Madewell JE, et al. Imaging bone metastases in breast cancer: techniques and recommendations for diagnosis. Lancet Oncol. 2009 Jun;10(6):606-14. PMID: 19482249.

9. Buijs M, Kamel IR, Vossen JA, et al. Assessment of metastatic breast cancer response to chemoembolization with contrast agent enhanced and diffusion-weighted MR imaging. J Vasc Interv Radiol. 2007 Aug;18(8):957-63. PMID: 17675611.

10. Cachin F, Prince HM, Hogg A, et al. Powerful prognostic stratification by [18F]fluorodeoxyglucose positron emission tomography in patients with metastatic breast cancer treated with high-dose chemotherapy. J Clin Oncol. 2006 Jul 1;24(19):3026-31. PMID: 16717291.

11. Cheng J, Lei L, Xu J, et al. 18F-fluoromisonidazole PET/CT: a potential tool for predicting primary endocrine therapy resistance in breast cancer. J Nucl Med. 2013 Mar;54(3):333-40. PMID: 23401605.

12. Contractor K, Aboagye EO, Jacob J, et al. Monitoring early response to taxane therapy in advanced breast cancer with circulating tumor cells and [(18)F] 3 -deoxy-3 -fluorothymidine PET: a pilot study. Biomark Med. 2012 Apr;6(2):231-3. PMID: 22448798.

13. Contractor KB, Kenny LM, Stebbing J, et al. [18F]-3'Deoxy-3'-fluorothymidine positron emission tomography and breast cancer response to docetaxel. Clin Cancer Res. 2011 Dec 15;17(24):7664-72. PMID: 22028493.

14. De Giorgi U, Valero V, Rohren E, et al. Circulating tumor cells and [18F]fluorodeoxyglucose positron emission tomography/computed tomography for outcome prediction in metastatic breast cancer. J Clin Oncol. 2009 Jul 10;27(20):3303-11. PMID: 19451443.

15. Dose Schwarz J, Bader M, Jenicke L, et al. Early prediction of response to chemotherapy in metastatic breast cancer using sequential 18F-FDG PET. J Nucl Med. 2005 Jul;46(7):1144-50. PMID: 16000283.

16. Haug AR, Tiega Donfack BP, Trumm C, et al. 18F-FDG PET/CT predicts survival after radioembolization of hepatic metastases from breast cancer. J Nucl Med. 2012 Mar;53(3):371-7. PMID: 22331219.

17. Huyge V, Garcia C, Alexiou J, et al. Heterogeneity of metabolic response to systemic therapy in metastatic breast cancer patients. Clin Oncol (R Coll Radiol). 2010 Dec;22(10):818-27. PMID: 20554438.

18. Kenny L, Coombes RC, Vigushin DM, et al. Imaging early changes in proliferation at 1 week post chemotherapy: a pilot study in breast cancer patients with 3'-deoxy-3'-[18F]fluorothymidine positron emission tomography. Eur J Nucl Med Mol Imaging. 2007 Sep;34(9):1339-47. PMID: 17333178.

19. Linden HM, Kurland BF, Peterson LM, et al. Fluoroestradiol positron emission tomography reveals differences in pharmacodynamics of aromatase inhibitors, tamoxifen, and fulvestrant in patients with metastatic breast cancer. Clin Cancer Res. 2011 Jul 15;17(14):4799-805. PMID: 21750198.

20. Linden HM, Stekhova SA, Link JM, et al. Quantitative fluoroestradiol positron emission tomography imaging predicts response to endocrine treatment in breast cancer. J Clin Oncol. 2006 Jun 20;24(18):2793-9. PMID: 16682724.

21. Mortazavi-Jehanno N, Giraudet AL, Champion L, et al. Assessment of response to endocrine therapy using FDG PET/CT in metastatic breast cancer: a pilot study. Eur J Nucl Med Mol Imaging. 2012 Mar;39(3):450-60. PMID: 22183107.

22. Pio BS, Park CK, Pietras R, et al. Usefulness of 3'-[F-18]fluoro-3'-deoxythymidine with positron emission tomography in predicting breast cancer response to therapy. Mol Imaging Biol. 2006 Jan-Feb;8(1):36-42. PMID: 16362149.

23. Specht JM, Tam SL, Kurland BF, et al. Serial 2-[18F] fluoro-2-deoxy-D-glucose positron emission tomography (FDG-PET) to monitor treatment of bone-dominant metastatic breast cancer predicts time to progression (TTP). Breast Cancer Res Treat. 2007 Sep;105(1):87-94. PMID: 17268819.

24. Tateishi U, Gamez C, Dawood S, et al. Bone metastases in patients with metastatic breast cancer: morphologic and metabolic monitoring of response to systemic therapy with integrated PET/CT. Radiology. 2008 Apr;247(1):189-96. PMID: 18372468.

25. Hayashi N, Costelloe CM, Hamaoka T, et al. A prospective study of bone tumor response assessment in metastatic breast cancer. Clin Breast Cancer. 2013 Feb;13(1):24-30. PMID: 23098575.

26. American College of Radiology Imaging Network. About Imaging Agents Or Tracers. 2013. www.acrin.org/PATIENTS/ABOUTIMAGINGEXAMSANDAGENTS/ABOUTIMAGINGAGENTSORTRACERS.aspx. Accessed November 6, 2013.

27. Gold LS, Klein G, Carr L, et al. The emergence of diagnostic imaging technologies in breast cancer: discovery, regulatory approval, reimbursement, and adoption in clinical guidelines. Cancer Imaging. 2012;12(1):13-24. PMID: 22275726.

28. Berger A. Magnetic resonance imaging. BMJ. 2002 Jan 5;324(7328):35. PMID: 11777806.

29. Li A, Wong CS, Wong MK, et al. Acute adverse reactions to magnetic resonance contrast media--gadolinium chelates. Br J Radiol. 2006 May;79(941):368-71. PMID: 16632615.

30. Robbins JB, Pozniak MA. Contrast Media Tutorial. Madison, WI: University of Wisconsin, Department of Radiology; 2010. www.radiology.wisc.edu/fileShelf/contrastCorner/files/ContrastAgentsTutorial.pdf. Accessed November 6 2013.

31. Podoloff D, Advani R, Allred C, et al. NCCN task force report: positron emission tomography (PET)/computed tomography (CT) scanning in cancer. J Natl Compr Canc Netw. 2007 May;5 Suppl 1:S1-S22; quiz S3-2. PMID: 17509259.

32. U.S. Food and Drug Administration. What are the Radiation Risks from CT? U.S. FDA; 2009. www.fda.gov/radiation-emittingproducts/radiationemittingproductsandprocedures/medicalimaging/medicalx-rays/ucm115329.htm. Accessed February 20 2014.

33. Zaidi H, Del Guerra A. An outlook on future design of hybrid PET/MRI systems. Medical physics. 2011;38:5667.

34. International Atomic Energy Agency. PET/CT Scanning. 2013. https://rpop.iaea.org/RPOP/RPoP/Content/InformationFor/HealthProfessionals/6_OtherClinicalSpecialities/PETCTscan.htm#PETCT_FAQ01. Accessed November 19 2013.

Acronyms and Abbreviations

BC	breast cancer
CA15-3	cancer antigen 15-3
CA27-29	cancer antigen 27-29
CEA	carcinoembryonic antigen
CT	computed tomography
CTC	circulating tumor cell
ER+	estrogen receptor positive
FDA	U.S. Food and Drug Administration
FDG	fluorodeoxyglucose
FDG-PET	fluorodeoxyglucose positron emission tomography
FES	fluoroestradiol
F-FMISO	F-fluoromisonidazole
FLT	fluorothymidine
GL	gray literature
HER2	Human Epidermal Growth Factor Receptor-2
KI	Key Informant
MBC	metastatic breast cancer
MRI	magnetic resonance imaging
NA	not applicable
NR	not reported
NSD	no significant difference
PET	positron emission tomography
PET/CT	positron emission tomography/ computed tomography
PET/MRI	positron emission tomography/magnetic resonance imaging
PL	published literature
SD	standard deviation
SPECT	single-photon emission computed tomography
SUV	standardized uptake value

Appendix A. Search Terms for Published Literature Review

Search #	Query	Number of Items Found
1	exp Diagnostic Imaging	1748368
2	exp Breast Neoplasms/dh, dt, pc, rt, su, th [Diet Therapy, Drug Therapy, Prevention & Control, Radiotherapy, Surgery, Therapy]	101694
3	exp Neoplasm Metastasis	158648
4	secondary.fs.	127910
5	(stag$ adj3 (four or iv)).mp. [mp=title, abstract, original title, name of substance word, subject heading word, keyword heading word, protocol supplementary concept, rare disease supplementary concept, unique identifier]	33298
6	3 or 4 or 5	286043
7	exp Prognosis	1108191
8	exp "Outcome and Process Assessment (Health Care)"	733807
9	exp Mortality	285802
10	mo.fs.	424456
11	exp survival analysis	192862
12	7 or 8	1173716
13	1 and 2 and 6 and 12	667
14	exp *Breast Neoplasms/dh, dt, pc, rt, su, th	65064
15	1 and 6 and 12 and 14	265
16	exp "Outcome Assessment (Health Care)"	710469
17	1 and 6 and 14 and 16	131
18	((treat$ or therap$ or interven$ or regimen$ or pharmacother$ or chemother$ or radiother$ or surger$ or surgic$) adj7 (effectiv$ or success$ or outcom$ or result$ or respons$ or reduc$ or remission$ or shrink$ or shrank or shrunk)).mp. [mp=title, abstract, original title, name of substance word, subject heading word, keyword heading word, protocol supplementary concept, rare disease supplementary concept, unique identifier]	1753900
19	1 and 6 and 14 and 18	297
20	19 not 17	166
21	Limit 20 to English language	114
22	((assess$ or determin$ or establish$ or confirm$ or evaluat$ or monitor$ or discover$ or determin$ or learn$ or discern$) adj7 (effectiv$ or success$ or outcom$ or result$ or respons$ or reduc$ or remission$ or shrink$ or shrank or shrunk)).mp.	963765
23	1 and 6 and 14 and 22	92
24	Limit 23 to English language	86
26	1 and 6 and 14 and 25	266
27	17 or 21 or 24 or 26	365
28	Limit 27 to yr="2003-Current"	256
29	Limit 28 to English language	197
30	Delete duplicates	158

Appendix B. Summary of Key Informant Interviews

What are the most commonly used imaging modalities to evaluate treatment of metastatic breast cancer?

- Choice of imaging strongly depends on where metastases are. If there are no boney metastases, would probably follow up with chest/abdomen/pelvis CT, but patients who had a baseline PET-CT are usually followed up with PET-CT also.
- MRI might be used on a patient with brain metastases, especially if they had a baseline scan.
- Most people use the Response Evaluation Criteria in Solid Tumors (RECIST) criteria to determine how well patients are responding to treatment, but the PET Response Criteria in Solid Tumors (PERCIST) is also used and may be more accurate.
- Use of PET-CT is extremely common because machines have been purchased and, once owned, might as well use them.

How often is imaging for treatment evaluation of metastatic breast cancer conducted?

- Usual assessment of metastatic disease involves a baseline PET-CT scan that could be repeated every 2-4 months, but if staging PET-CT is not covered by insurance, a bone scan or chest/abdomen/pelvis CT (or both) are often used.
- Imaging may be avoided if patient is displaying symptoms.
- The choice of imaging and intervals are often dictated by insurance coverage. PET-CT is not covered earlier than 2 month followup. Also, some plans require potentially time-consuming peer-to-peer discussions about whether PET-CT is warranted, so that discourages doctors from ordering it.
- Intervals of imaging depend on treatment cycles. Also, unlikely to see clinical progression before 2-3 months of treatment so most imaging is not ordered earlier than that.
- Patients can also experience anxiety about imaging so that's a reason to limit tests, but on the other hand, if tests show treatment is working, that is very heartening for patients.

When is PET-CT used versus bone scan?

- At baseline, PET-CT tends to find more lesions than bone scan; this usually doesn't affect treatment choice unless a bone lesion is found, since treating bone lesions has large effect on the patient's quality of life.
- PET-CT can help visualize followup of disease in difficult to visualize areas, such as nodes, or if anatomic alterations have occurred to the patient as a results of treatment.

Which imaging modalities are being over/under utilized?

- PET-CT probably less appropriately utilized because it is a newer technology. This is an active area of research.
- Some imaging is driven by pharmaceutical trials that dictate certain types of followup. This tends to become a familiar/usual approach in practice.

Differences in imaging use between academic versus community settings?

- Community practice seems to be more variable.
- Patient preparation and physician interpretation is often inferior in the community setting.
- Patient insurance status might come into play more often in community setting, e.g., patient without adequate insurance might be steered toward less expensive imaging.
- Physicians in academic settings may feel more pressure to use the most recent (and therefore most expensive) technologies. May have a greater fear of lawsuits if they fail to order a test.

What policies do payers put in place to influence use of imaging for treatment evaluation of metastatic breast cancer?

- Payers use Radiology Benefit Managers (RBMs) to encourage providers to minimize use of imaging, but not a lot of evidence behind their decisions.
- Payers require peer-to-peer consultations. Often does discourage imaging from being ordered but again, unclear whether this is appropriate.

How are decisions to purchase imaging equipment used to evaluate treatment for metastatic breast cancer made?

- Most cancer centers have CT and PET-CT because they are used for many cancers and they want to promote themselves as having the latest and greatest technology to attract patients.

What types of imaging is most commonly reimbursed for treatment evaluation of metastatic breast cancer? What are the advantages and disadvantages of these types of imaging?

- CT and PET-CT pretty readily reimbursed. For other types of imaging, depends where the metastases are, e.g. if a woman has liver metastases, liver ultrasound would be readily reimbursed.
- The frequency of imaging is variable among payers.
- Patient anxiety: sometimes imaging is useful for reassuring the patient, but other times waiting for the results is very stressful for them.

Other guidelines used to determine choice of imaging besides NCCN?

- No. Even NCCN guidelines concluded there was not enough data to make suggestions about use of imaging for assessing response to therapy.
- NCCN guidelines heavily influenced by medical oncologists and other nonimagers.

Do accreditation programs influence the type of imaging chosen?

- For devices, the American College of Radiology (ACR) provides accreditation. Most centers maintain that accreditation, but it does not cover patient preparation, which is important.
- No accreditation for who reads PET-CT scans. Guidelines for minimum training to read scans exist but are not enforced.
- Even at major cancer centers, only 10 percent of PET-CTs done in a facility would be related to breast cancer so difficult for physicians at smaller centers to gain experience interpreting breast images.

What is the role of patient choice?

- Patient preferences usually push clinicians to do more tests and more expensive tests.
- For some physicians, it is easier to just order a test than take the time to argue about it with patients.
- Patients usually don't want to reduce their imaging. For example, once they have had PET-CT, they don't want to only CT.
- Patients often don't have tests explained to them, particularly the pros/cons, etc. Patients don't get enough information about the reasons for tests, what they mean, etc. because person interpreting scans rarely interacts with patient. They get much better explanations about treatment.
- Patients don't grasp the use of tests, their accuracy, interpretation, etc. Their research about their disease tends to focus on treatment.
- Patients often willing to take extreme risks to avoid the smallest chance of dying of breast cancer.

What factors related to imaging are most important to patients?

- Patients often do not realize several imaging modalities exist and they have options.
- Patients expect their tests to show them if treatment has been successful.
- Out-of-pocket expenses vary: patients who have good insurance coverage or Medicaid generally don't think about costs but patients with other types of insurance often have high copays and deductibles, requiring them to make decisions based on cost rather than what's best for their health.
- Many patients reach out-of-pocket maximum because of expense of treatment so during treatment are usually not concerned about out-of-pocket costs.
- Some patients have claustrophobia or reactions to contrast when receiving imaging, but in general the discomfort from imaging is much easier to tolerate than that from treatment.
- Imagers generally do not interact with patients. Communication is directed to the referring physicians but they don't necessarily communicate information about the images as well as the imager might.
- Patients discuss the inconvenience of tests, especially PET since it involves long idle periods of time needed to allow radiotracer circulation.
- A lot of imaging reassures patients (not a trivial issue) but provides no clinical benefit. Alternative ways to reassure patient might be less expensive and potentially have fewer risks.
- Patients discuss which imaging facilities are the most comfortable and offer them the most perks (e.g. warm blankets and herbal tea).
- Most patients do not consider the accuracy of imaging tests and usually do not research imaging on their own the way they research treatment options.

What emerging technologies can we expect in next 5 years or so?

- PET-MRI might become relevant for brain metastases because MR does a better job imaging the brain than CT.
- Emerging data show that if tests are done in a certain order, patient may avoid some (e.g. PET can obviate the need for a bone scan).

- Imaging with PET using 18F-fluoroestradiol (FES) as a tracer, may be available in 3-5 years.
- Patients would prefer blood test over imaging if it were accurate.
- So far for breast cancer, tumor markers and circulating malignant cells in blood samples are unreliable tests because breast cancer is such a heterogeneous disease. Hopefully in the next 10-15 years these tests will have improved so much that they will drastically curtail imaging.
- Quantitative assessment of treatment response using standard uptake value changes seen on FDG-PET after the first course of treatment would allow clinicians to know how the tumors are responding so they could adjust the doses of chemotherapies. Further research is needed before associations could be validated and reproducible.

What are some important research needs?

- New tracers for PET imaging
- Accurate tumor markers that could show whether patient is responding to treatment using a blood test instead of imaging.
- No studies of long-term outcomes. Do these technologies actually change outcomes, quality of life, or treatment selection? Current studies are generally single center, no clinical outcomes (especially long term). These could be embedded in therapeutic trials.
- Studies of communication with patients. The most knowledgeable person (the one interpreting the image) is often not available to patients for questions, especially in nonacademic settings.
- Studies that allow better understanding of tumor biology.
- Imaging technologies that identify smallest tumors possible to reduce breast cancer recurrence.
- Imaging that is more specific to each patient's type of cancer so a particular tumor could be characterized by the genetic or even proteomic level and then treated without damaging healthy tissue.
- Increased accuracy is needed to make a better treatment decisions.
- Use of imaging to evaluate side effects of treatment, e.g., women taking Herceptin (which can affect cardiac function) might have better outcomes if they received echocardiography during their treatment to determine whether their heart function was being affected. If it were, they could be put on medications that would minimize cardiac side effects. Most imaging currently focuses solely on the cancer and metastases, rather than other parts of the body that might be affected by toxic treatments.
- After baseline scan, how often should imaging be repeated?

What are barriers that inhibit research on imaging for treatment evaluation for metastatic breast cancer?

- New technologies are not used if there is no reimbursement for development.
- Regulatory barriers also exist. Time and cost for approval may deter development of product.

Appendix C. List of Abstracted Published Literature Studies

Number	Citation
1	Buijs M, Kamel IR, Vossen JA, et al. Assessment of metastatic breast cancer response to chemoembolization with contrast agent enhanced and diffusion-weighted MR imaging. J Vasc Interv Radiol. 18(8):957-63, 2007 Aug. PMID: 17675611.
2	Cachin F, Prince HM, Hogg A, et al. Powerful prognostic stratification by [18F]fluorodeoxyglucose positron emission tomography in patients with metastatic breast cancer treated with high-dose chemotherapy. J Clin Oncol. 24(19):3026-31, 2006 Jul 1. PMID: 16717291.
3	Cheng J, Lei L., Xu J, et al. 18F-fluoromisonidazole PET/CT: a potential tool for predicting primary endocrine therapy resistance in breast cancer. J Nucl Med. 54(3):333-40, 2013 Mar. PMID: 23401605.
4	Contractor KB, Kenny LM, Stebbing J, et al. [18F]-3'Deoxy-3'-fluorothymidine positron emission tomography and breast cancer response to docetaxel. Clin Cancer Res. 17(24):7664-72, 2011 Dec 15. PMID: 22028493.
5	Contractor K, Aboagye EO, Jacob J, et al. Monitoring early response to taxane therapy in advanced breast cancer with circulating tumor cells and [(18)F] 3`-deoxy-3`-fluorothymidine PET: a pilot study. Biomark Med. 6(2):231-3, 2012 Apr. PMID: 22448798 .
6	De Giorgi U, Valero V, Rohren E, et al. Fritsche HA. Macapinlac HA. Hortobagyi GN. Cristofanilli M. Circulating tumor cells and [18F]fluorodeoxyglucose positron emission tomography/computed tomography for outcome prediction in metastatic breast cancer. J Clin Oncol 27 (20) 3303-11, 2009. PMID: 19451443.
7	Dose Schwarz J, Bader M, Jenicke L, et al. Early prediction of response to chemotherapy in metastatic breast cancer using sequential 18F-FDG PET. J Nucl Med. 46(7):1144-50, 2005 Jul. PMID: 16000283.
8	Haug AR, Tiega Donfack BP, Trumm C., et al. Bartenstein P. Heinemann V. Hacker M. 18F-FDG PET/CT predicts survival after radioembolization of hepatic metastases from breast cancer. J Nucl Med. 53(3):371-7, 2012 Mar. PMID: 22331219.
9	Huyge V, Garcia C, Alexiou J, eet al. Heterogeneity of metabolic response to systemic therapy in metastatic breast cancer patients. Clin Oncol (R Coll Radiol). 22(10):818-27, 2010 Dec. PMID: 20554438.
10	Kenny L, Coombes RC, Vigushin DM, et al. Imaging early changes in proliferation at 1 week post chemotherapy: a pilot study in breast cancer patients with 3'-deoxy-3'-[18F]fluorothymidine positron emission tomography. Eur J Nucl Med Mol Imaging. 34(9):1339-47, 2007 Sep. PMID: 17333178.
11	Linden HM, Stekhova SA, Link JM, et al. Quantitative fluoroestradiol positron emission tomography imaging predicts response to endocrine treatment in breast cancer. J Clin Oncol. 24(18):2793-9, 2006 Jun 20. PMID: 16682724.
12	Linden HM, Kurland BF, Peterson LM, et al. Fluoroestradiol positron emission tomography reveals differences in pharmacodynamics of aromatase inhibitors, tamoxifen, and fulvestrant in patients with metastatic breast cancer. Clin Cancer Res. 17(14):4799-805, 2011 Jul 15. PMID: 21750198.
13	Mortazavi-Jehanno N, Giraudet AL, Champion L et al. Assessment of response to endocrine therapy using FDG PET/CT in metastatic breast cancer: a pilot study. Eur J Nucl Med Mol Imaging. 39(3):450-60, 2012 Mar. PMID: 22183107.
14	Pio BS, Park CK, Pietras R, et al. Usefulness of 3'-[F-18]fluoro-3'-deoxythymidine with positron emission tomography in predicting breast cancer response to therapy. Mol Imaging Biol 8 (1) 36-42, 2006. PMID: 16362149.
15	Specht JM, Tam SL, Kurland BF, et al. Serial 2-[18F] fluoro-2-deoxy-D-glucose positron emission tomography (FDG-PET) to monitor treatment of bone-dominant metastatic breast cancer predicts time to progression (TTP). Breast Cancer Res Treat 105 (1) 2007. PMID: 17268819.
16	Tateishi U, Gamez C, Dawood S, et al. Bone metastases in patients with metastatic breast cancer: morphologic and metabolic monitoring of response to systemic therapy with integrated PET/CT. Radiology. 247, 2008. PMID: 18372468.
17	Hayashi N, Costelloe CM, Hamaoka T, et al. A prospective study of bone tumor response assessment in metastatic breast cancer. Clin Breast Cancer. 2013 Feb;13(1):24-30. PMID: 23098575.

Appendix D. List of Excluded Published Literature Studies

Number	Citation	Reason for Exclusion
1	Agarwal A, Munoz-Najar U, Klueh U, et al. N-acetyl-cysteine promotes angiostatin production and vascular collapse in an orthotopic model of breast cancer. Am J Pathol. 2004 May;164(5):1683-96. PMID: 15111315.	Article did not address use of imaging for treatment evaluation for metastatic breast cancer.
2	Akazawa K, Tamaki Y, Taguchi T, et al. Potential of reduction in total tumor volume measured with 3D-MRI as a prognostic factor for locally-advanced breast cancer patients treated with primary chemotherapy. Breast J. 2008 Nov-Dec;14(6):523-31. PMID: 19000056.	Article did not include metastatic breast cancer patients.
3	Ali AM, Ueno T, Tanaka S, et al. Determining circulating endothelial cells using CellSearch system during preoperative systemic chemotherapy in breast cancer patients. Eur J Cancer. 2011 Oct;47(15):2265-72. PMID: 21737256.	Article did not address use of imaging for treatment evaluation for metastatic breast cancer.
4	Altenburg JD, Siddiqui RA. Omega-3 polyunsaturated fatty acids down-modulate CXCR4 expression and function in MDA-MB-231 breast cancer cells. Mol Cancer Res. 2009 Jul;7(7):1013-20. PMID: 19567784.	Article did not address use of imaging for treatment evaluation for metastatic breast cancer.
5	Apple SK, Matin M, Olsen EP, et al. Significance of lobular intraepithelial neoplasia at margins of breast conservation specimens: a report of 38 cases and literature review. Diagn Pathol. 2010;5:54. PMID: 20727142.	Article did not address use of imaging for treatment evaluation for metastatic breast cancer.
6	Asakura H, Takashima H, Mitani M, et al. Unknown primary carcinoma, diagnosed as inflammatory breast cancer,and successfully treated with trastuzumab and vinorelbine. Int J Clin Oncol. 2005 Aug;10(4):285-8. PMID: 16136377.	Article did not address use of imaging for treatment evaluation for metastatic breast cancer.
7	Bangash AK, Atassi B, Kaklamani V, et al. 90Y radioembolization of metastatic breast cancer to the liver: toxicity, imaging response, survival. J Vasc Interv Radiol. 2007 May;18(5):621-8. PMID: 17494843.	Article did not address use of imaging for treatment evaluation for metastatic breast cancer.
8	Barth RJ, Jr., Gibson GR, Carney PA, et al. Detection of breast cancer on screening mammography allows patients to be treated with less-toxic therapy. AJR Am J Roentgenol. 2005 Jan;184(1):324-9. PMID: 15615996.	Article did not address use of imaging for treatment evaluation for metastatic breast cancer.
9	Bauerle T, Bartling S, Berger M, et al. Imaging anti-angiogenic treatment response with DCE-VCT, DCE-MRI and DWI in an animal model of breast cancer bone metastasis. Eur J Radiol. 2010 Feb;73(2):280-7. PMID: 19070445.	Non-human study.
10	Bauerle T, Hilbig H, Bartling S, et al. Bevacizumab inhibits breast cancer-induced osteolysis, surrounding soft tissue metastasis, and angiogenesis in rats as visualized by VCT and MRI. Neoplasia. 2008 May;10(5):511-20. PMID: 18472968.	Non-human study.
11	Biersack HJ, Bender H, Palmedo H. FDG-PET in monitoring therapy of breast cancer. Eur J Nucl Med Mol Imaging. 2004 Jun;31 Suppl 1:S112-7. PMID: 15112111.	Review article. Reviewed citations for additional relevant articles.
12	Boccardo FM, Casabona F, Friedman D, et al. Surgical prevention of arm lymphedema after breast cancer treatment. Ann Surg Oncol. 2011 Sep;18(9):2500-5. PMID: 21369739.	Article did not address use of imaging for treatment evaluation for metastatic breast cancer.
13	Bondareva A, Downey CM, Ayres F, et al. The lysyl oxidase inhibitor, beta-aminopropionitrile, diminishes the metastatic colonization potential of circulating breast cancer cells. PLoS One. 2009;4(5):e5620. PMID: 19440335.	Article did not address use of imaging for treatment evaluation for metastatic breast cancer.
14	Bricou A, Duval MA, Charon Y, et al. Mobile gamma cameras in breast cancer care - a review. Eur J Surg Oncol. 2013 May;39(5):409-16. PMID: 23465183.	Article did not address use of imaging for treatment evaluation for metastatic breast cancer.

Number	Citation	Reason for Exclusion
15	Brown-Glaberman U, Graham A, Stopeck A. A case of metaplastic carcinoma of the breast responsive to chemotherapy with Ifosfamide and Etoposide: improved antitumor response by targeting sarcomatous features. Breast J. 2010 Nov-Dec;16(6):663-5. PMID: 21070449.	Article did not address use of imaging for treatment evaluation for metastatic breast cancer.
16	Bullitt E, Lin NU, Ewend MG, et al. Tumor therapeutic response and vessel tortuosity: preliminary report in metastatic breast cancer. Med Image Comput Comput Assist Interv. 2006;9(Pt 2):561-8. PMID: 17354817.	Article did not address use of imaging for treatment evaluation for metastatic breast cancer.
17	Burkholder HC, Witherspoon LE, Burns RP, et al. Breast surgery techniques: preoperative bracketing wire localization by surgeons. Am Surg. 2007 Jun;73(6):574-8; discussion 8-9. PMID: 17658094.	Article did not address use of imaging for treatment evaluation for metastatic breast cancer.
18	Caralt M, Bilbao I, Cortes J, et al. Hepatic resection for liver metastases as part of the "oncosurgical" treatment of metastatic breast cancer. Ann Surg Oncol. 2008 Oct;15(10):2804-10. PMID: 18670821.	Article did not address use of imaging for treatment evaluation for metastatic breast cancer.
19	Castro Pena P, Kirova YM, Campana F, et al. Anatomical, clinical and radiological delineation of target volumes in breast cancer radiotherapy planning: individual variability, questions and answers. Br J Radiol. 2009 Jul;82(979):595-9. PMID: 19255114.	Article did not address use of imaging for treatment evaluation for metastatic breast cancer.
20	Chen JH, Mehta RS, Nalcioglu O, et al. Inflammatory breast cancer after neoadjuvant chemotherapy: can magnetic resonance imaging precisely diagnose the final pathological response? Ann Surg Oncol. 2008 Dec;15(12):3609-13. PMID: 18807091.	Article about diagnostic breast imaging, not imaging for treatment evaluation.
21	Cheung YC, Chen SC, Ueng SH, et al. Dynamic enhanced computed tomography values of locally advanced breast cancers predicting axilla nodal metastasis after neoadjuvant chemotherapy. J Comput Assist Tomogr. 2009 May-Jun;33(3):422-5. PMID: 19478638.	Article did not address use of imaging for treatment evaluation for metastatic breast cancer.
22	Conrado-Abrao F, Das-Neves-Pereira JC, Fernandes A, et al. Thoracoscopic approach in the treatment of breast cancer relapse in the internal mammary lymph node. Interact Cardiovasc Thorac Surg. 2010 Sep;11(3):328-30. PMID: 20576656.	Article did not address use of imaging for treatment evaluation for metastatic breast cancer.
23	Dalus K, Reitsamer R, Holzmannhofer J, et al. Lymphoscintigraphy in breast cancer patients after neoadjuvant chemotherapy. Diagnostic value and the work-up of sentinel node negative patients. Nuklearmedizin. 2011;50(1):33-8. PMID: 21336417.	Article did not address use of imaging for treatment evaluation for metastatic breast cancer.
24	De Los Santos J, Bernreuter W, Keene K, et al. Accuracy of breast magnetic resonance imaging in predicting pathologic response in patients treated with neoadjuvant chemotherapy. Clin Breast Cancer. 2011 Oct;11(5):312-9. PMID: 21831721.	Article did not include metastatic breast cancer patients.
25	Donadio M, Ardine M, Berruti A, et al. Weekly cisplatin plus capecitabine in metastatic breast cancer patients heavily pretreated with both anthracycline and taxanes. Oncology. 2005;69(5):408-13. PMID: 16319512.	Article did not address use of imaging for treatment evaluation for metastatic breast cancer.
26	Driul L, Bernardi S, Bertozzi S, et al. New surgical trends in breast cancer treatment: conservative interventions and oncoplastic breast surgery. Minerva Ginecol. 2013 Jun;65(3):289-96. PMID: 23689171.	Article did not address use of imaging for treatment evaluation for metastatic breast cancer.
27	Dunnwald LK, Gralow JR, Ellis GK, et al. Tumor metabolism and blood flow changes by positron emission tomography: relation to survival in patients treated with neoadjuvant chemotherapy for locally advanced breast cancer. J Clin Oncol. 2008 Sep 20;26(27):4449-57. PMID: 18626006.	Article did not include metastatic breast cancer patients.
28	El-Mabhouh AA, Nation PN, Abele JT, et al. A conjugate of gemcitabine with bisphosphonate (Gem/BP) shows potential as a targeted bone-specific therapeutic agent in an animal model of human breast cancer bone metastases. Oncol Res. 2011;19(6):287-95. PMID: 21776824.	Article did not address use of imaging for treatment evaluation for metastatic breast cancer.
29	Eubank WB, Mankoff DA. Evolving role of positron emission tomography in breast cancer imaging. Semin Nucl Med. 2005 Apr;35(2):84-99. PMID: 15765372.	Review article. Reviewed citations for additional relevant articles.

Number	Citation	Reason for Exclusion
30	Fanale MA, Uyei AR, Theriault RL, et al. Treatment of metastatic breast cancer with trastuzumab and vinorelbine during pregnancy. Clin Breast Cancer. 2005 Oct;6(4):354-6. PMID: 16277887.	Article did not address use of imaging for treatment evaluation for metastatic breast cancer.
31	Fischer U, Baum F, Luftner-Nagel S. Preoperative MR imaging in patients with breast cancer: preoperative staging, effects on recurrence rates, and outcome analysis. Magn Reson Imaging Clin N Am. 2006 Aug;14(3):351-62, vi. PMID: 17098176.	Article did not address use of imaging for treatment evaluation for metastatic breast cancer.
32	Fong S, Itahana Y, Sumida T, et al. Id-1 as a molecular target in therapy for breast cancer cell invasion and metastasis. Proc Natl Acad Sci U S A. 2003 Nov 11;100(23):13543-8. PMID: 14578451.	Article did not address use of imaging for treatment evaluation for metastatic breast cancer.
33	Gatcombe HG, Olson TA, Esiashvili N. Metastatic primary angiosarcoma of the breast in a pediatric patient with a complete response to systemic chemotherapy and definitive radiation therapy: case report and review of the literature. J Pediatr Hematol Oncol. 2010 Apr;32(3):192-4. PMID: 20186104.	Article did not address use of imaging for treatment evaluation for metastatic breast cancer.
34	Gennari A, Piccardo A, Altrinetti V, et al. Whither the PET scan? The role of PET imaging in the staging and treatment of breast cancer. Curr Oncol Rep. 2012 Feb;14(1):20-6. PMID: 22094933.	Review article. Reviewed citations for additional relevant articles.
35	Gerber B, Heintze K, Stubert J, et al. Axillary lymph node dissection in early-stage invasive breast cancer: is it still standard today? Breast Cancer Res Treat. 2011 Aug;128(3):613-24. PMID: 21523451.	Article did not address use of imaging for treatment evaluation for metastatic breast cancer.
36	Giacalone PL, Bourdon A, Trinh PD, et al. Radioguided occult lesion localization plus sentinel node biopsy (SNOLL) versus wire-guided localization plus sentinel node detection: a case control study of 129 unifocal pure invasive non-palpable breast cancers. Eur J Surg Oncol. 2012 Mar;38(3):222-9. PMID: 22231127.	Article did not address use of imaging for treatment evaluation for metastatic breast cancer.
37	Giglio P, Tremont-Lukats IW, Groves MD. Response of neoplastic meningitis from solid tumors to oral capecitabine. J Neurooncol. 2003 Nov;65(2):167-72. PMID: 14686737.	Article did not address use of imaging for treatment evaluation for metastatic breast cancer.
38	Gilardi L, Paganelli G. Is a SUV cut-off necessary in the evaluation of the response of axillary lymph node metastases to neoadjuvant therapy? Eur J Nucl Med Mol Imaging. 2010 Nov;37(11):2202. PMID: 20821210.	Letter to the editor.
39	Goldoni S, Seidler DG, Heath J, et al. An antimetastatic role for decorin in breast cancer. Am J Pathol. 2008 Sep;173(3):844-55. PMID: 18688028.	Article did not address use of imaging for treatment evaluation for metastatic breast cancer.
40	Goyal S, Puri T, Julka PK, et al. Excellent response to letrozole in brain metastases from breast cancer. Acta Neurochir (Wien). 2008 Jun;150(6):613-4; discussion 4-5. PMID: 18458809.	Article did not address use of imaging for treatment evaluation for metastatic breast cancer.
41	Grabau D, Dihge L, Ferno M, et al. Completion axillary dissection can safely be omitted in screen detected breast cancer patients with micrometastases. A decade's experience from a single institution. Eur J Surg Oncol. 2013 Jun;39(6):601-7. PMID: 23579175.	Article did not address use of imaging for treatment evaluation for metastatic breast cancer.
42	Gralow JR, Biermann JS, Farooki A, et al. NCCN Task Force Report: Bone Health in Cancer Care. J Natl Compr Canc Netw. 2009 Jun;7 Suppl 3:S1-32; quiz S3-5. PMID: 19555589.	Article did not address use of imaging for treatment evaluation for metastatic breast cancer.
43	Hayashi H, Kimura M, Yoshimoto N, et al. A case of HER2-positive male breast cancer with lung metastases showing a good response to trastuzumab and paclitaxel treatment. Breast Cancer. 2009;16(2):136-40. PMID: 18548321.	Article did not address use of imaging for treatment evaluation for metastatic breast cancer.
44	Hill KL, Jr., Lipson AC, Sheehan JM. Brain magnetic resonance imaging changes after sorafenib and sunitinib chemotherapy in patients with advanced renal cell and breast carcinoma. J Neurosurg. 2009 Sep;111(3):497-503. PMID: 19199506.	Article did not address use of imaging for treatment evaluation for metastatic breast cancer.

Number	Citation	Reason for Exclusion
45	Hiraga T, Williams PJ, Ueda A, et al. Zoledronic acid inhibits visceral metastases in the 4T1/luc mouse breast cancer model. Clin Cancer Res. 2004 Jul 1;10(13):4559-67. PMID: 15240548.	Article did not address use of imaging for treatment evaluation for metastatic breast cancer.
46	Hsiang DJ, Yamamoto M, Mehta RS, et al. Predicting nodal status using dynamic contrast-enhanced magnetic resonance imaging in patients with locally advanced breast cancer undergoing neoadjuvant chemotherapy with and without sequential trastuzumab. Arch Surg. 2007 Sep;142(9):855-61; discussion 60-1. PMID: 17875840.	Article did not include metastatic breast cancer patients.
47	Hu Z, Gerseny H, Zhang Z, et al. Oncolytic adenovirus expressing soluble TGFbeta receptor II-Fc-mediated inhibition of established bone metastases: a safe and effective systemic therapeutic approach for breast cancer. Mol Ther. 2011 Sep;19(9):1609-18. PMID: 21712815.	Article did not address use of imaging for treatment evaluation for metastatic breast cancer.
48	Hua F, Feng X, Guan Y, et al. Non-Hodgkin's lymphoma of supraclavicular lymph nodes can mimic metastasis of breast cancer during chemotherapy on FDG PET/CT. Clin Nucl Med. 2009 Sep;34(9):594-5. PMID: 19692820.	Article did not address use of imaging for treatment evaluation for metastatic breast cancer.
49	Huyn ST, Burton JB, Sato M, et al. A potent, imaging adenoviral vector driven by the cancer-selective mucin-1 promoter that targets breast cancer metastasis. Clin Cancer Res. 2009 May 1;15(9):3126-34. PMID: 19366829.	Article did not address use of imaging for treatment evaluation for metastatic breast cancer.
50	Intra M, Trifiro G, Viale G, et al. Second biopsy of axillary sentinel lymph node for reappearing breast cancer after previous sentinel lymph node biopsy. Ann Surg Oncol. 2005 Nov;12(11):895-9. PMID: 16195833.	Article did not address use of imaging for treatment evaluation for metastatic breast cancer.
51	Isola V, Pece A, Pierro L. Photodynamic therapy with verteporfin of choroidal malignancy from breast cancer. Am J Ophthalmol. 2006 Nov;142(5):885-7. PMID: 17056382.	Article did not address use of imaging for treatment evaluation for metastatic breast cancer.
52	Javid S, Segara D, Lotfi P, et al. Can breast MRI predict axillary lymph node metastasis in women undergoing neoadjuvant chemotherapy. Ann Surg Oncol. 2010 Jul;17(7):1841-6. PMID: 20143266.	Article about diagnostic breast imaging, not imaging for treatment evaluation.
53	Jones MD, Liu JC, Barthel TK, et al. A proteasome inhibitor, bortezomib, inhibits breast cancer growth and reduces osteolysis by downregulating metastatic genes. Clin Cancer Res. 2010 Oct 15;16(20):4978-89. PMID: 20843837.	Article did not address use of imaging for treatment evaluation for metastatic breast cancer.
54	Jones RL, Berry GJ, Rubens RD, et al. Clinical and pathological absence of cardiotoxicity after liposomal doxorubicin. Lancet Oncol. 2004 Sep;5(9):575-7. PMID: 15337488.	Article did not address use of imaging for treatment evaluation for metastatic breast cancer.
55	Kaliki S, Shields CL, Al-Dahmash SA, et al. Photodynamic therapy for choroidal metastasis in 8 cases. Ophthalmology. 2012 Jun;119(6):1218-22. PMID: 22386261.	Article did not address use of imaging for treatment evaluation for metastatic breast cancer.
56	Katalinic D, Stern-Padovan R, Ivanac I, et al. Symptomatic cardiac metastases of breast cancer 27 years after mastectomy: a case report with literature review--pathophysiology of molecular mechanisms and metastatic pathways, clinical aspects, diagnostic procedures and treatment modalities. World J Surg Oncol. 2013;11:14. PMID: 23343205.	Article did not address use of imaging for treatment evaluation for metastatic breast cancer.
57	Kelemen G, Uhercsak G, Ormandi K, et al. Long-term efficiency and toxicity of adjuvant dose-dense sequential adriamycin-Paclitaxel-cyclophosphamide chemotherapy in high-risk breast cancer. Oncology. 2010;78(3-4):271-3. PMID: 20523088.	Article did not address use of imaging for treatment evaluation for metastatic breast cancer.
58	Khalili P, Arakelian A, Chen G, et al. A non-RGD-based integrin binding peptide (ATN-161) blocks breast cancer growth and metastasis in vivo. Mol Cancer Ther. 2006 Sep;5(9):2271-80. PMID: 16985061.	Article did not address use of imaging for treatment evaluation for metastatic breast cancer.

Number	Citation	Reason for Exclusion
59	Kilbride KE, Lee MC, Nees AV, et al. Axillary staging prior to neoadjuvant chemotherapy for breast cancer: predictors of recurrence. Ann Surg Oncol. 2008 Nov;15(11):3252-8. PMID: 18784961.	Article did not address use of imaging for treatment evaluation for metastatic breast cancer.
60	Kinhikar RA, Deshpande SS, Mahantshetty U, et al. HDR brachytherapy combined with 3-D conformal vs. IMRT in left-sided breast cancer patients including internal mammary chain: comparative analysis of dosimetric and technical parameters. J Appl Clin Med Phys. 2005 Summer;6(3):1-12. PMID: 16143787.	Article did not address use of imaging for treatment evaluation for metastatic breast cancer.
61	Kodack DP, Chung E, Yamashita H, et al. Combined targeting of HER2 and VEGFR2 for effective treatment of HER2-amplified breast cancer brain metastases. Proc Natl Acad Sci U S A. 2012 Nov 6;109(45):E3119-27. PMID: 23071298.	Article did not address use of imaging for treatment evaluation for metastatic breast cancer.
62	Koehler KE, Ohlinger R. Sensitivity and specificity of preoperative ultrasonography for diagnosing nodal metastases in patients with breast cancer. Ultraschall Med. 2011 Aug;32(4):393-9. PMID: 20938895.	Article did not address use of imaging for treatment evaluation for metastatic breast cancer.
63	Kogure K, Sakurai T, Tsuzuki Y, et al. Long-term survival after hepatectomy for large metastatic breast cancer: a case report. Hepatogastroenterology. 2003 May-Jun;50(51):827-9. PMID: 12828095.	Article did not address use of imaging for treatment evaluation for metastatic breast cancer.
64	Kokke MC, Jannink I, Barneveld PC, et al. Incidence of axillary recurrence in 113 sentinel node negative breast cancer patients: a 3-year follow-up study. Eur J Surg Oncol. 2005 Apr;31(3):221-5. PMID: 15780554.	Article did not address use of imaging for treatment evaluation for metastatic breast cancer.
65	Koolen BB, Valdes Olmos RA, Elkhuizen PH, et al. Locoregional lymph node involvement on 18F-FDG PET/CT in breast cancer patients scheduled for neoadjuvant chemotherapy. Breast Cancer Res Treat. 2012 Aug;135(1):231-40. PMID: 22872522.	Article about diagnostic breast imaging, not imaging for treatment evaluation.
66	Kothari MS, Rusby JE, Agusti AA, et al. Sentinel lymph node biopsy after previous axillary surgery: A review. Eur J Surg Oncol. 2012 Jan;38(1):8-15. PMID: 22032909.	Article did not address use of imaging for treatment evaluation for metastatic breast cancer.
67	Krainick-Strobel UE, Lichtenegger W, Wallwiener D, et al. Neoadjuvant letrozole in postmenopausal estrogen and/or progesterone receptor positive breast cancer: a phase IIb/III trial to investigate optimal duration of preoperative endocrine therapy. BMC Cancer. 2008;8:62. PMID: 18302747.	Article did not address use of imaging for treatment evaluation for metastatic breast cancer.
68	Krak NC, Hoekstra OS, Lammertsma AA. Measuring response to chemotherapy in locally advanced breast cancer: methodological considerations. Eur J Nucl Med Mol Imaging. 2004 Jun;31 Suppl 1:S103-11. PMID: 15103507.	Article did not include metastatic breast cancer patients.
69	Krukemeyer MG, Wagner W, Jakobs M, et al. Tumor regression by means of magnetic drug targeting. Nanomedicine (Lond). 2009 Dec;4(8):875-82. PMID: 19958224.	Article did not address use of imaging for treatment evaluation for metastatic breast cancer.
70	Kubota K, Ogawa Y, Nishigawa T, et al. Tissue harmonic imaging sonography of the axillary lymph nodes: evaluation of response to neoadjuvant chemotherapy in breast cancer patients. Oncol Rep. 2003 Nov-Dec;10(6):1911-4. PMID: 14534717.	Article did not address use of imaging for treatment evaluation for metastatic breast cancer.
71	Kumar R, Alavi A. Fluorodeoxyglucose-PET in the management of breast cancer. Radiol Clin North Am. 2004 Nov;42(6):1113-22, ix. PMID: 15488561.	Article did not address use of imaging for treatment evaluation for metastatic breast cancer.
72	Labidi SI, Bachelot T, Ray-Coquard I, et al. Bevacizumab and paclitaxel for breast cancer patients with central nervous system metastases: a case series. Clin Breast Cancer. 2009 May;9(2):118-21. PMID: 19433393.	Article did not address use of imaging for treatment evaluation for metastatic breast cancer.

Number	Citation	Reason for Exclusion
73	Latif N, Rana F, Guthrie T. Breast cancer and HIV in the era of highly active antiretroviral therapy: two case reports and review of the literature. Breast J. 2011 Jan-Feb;17(1):87-92. PMID: 21134040.	Article did not address use of imaging for treatment evaluation for metastatic breast cancer.
74	Leonard GD, Swain SM. Ductal carcinoma in situ, complexities and challenges. J Natl Cancer Inst. 2004 Jun 16;96(12):906-20. PMID: 15199110.	Article did not address use of imaging for treatment evaluation for metastatic breast cancer.
75	Leung JW. Screening mammography reduces morbidity of breast cancer treatment. AJR Am J Roentgenol. 2005 May;184(5):1508-9. PMID: 15855106.	Article did not address use of imaging for treatment evaluation for metastatic breast cancer.
76	Li X, Ferrel GL, Guerra MC, et al. Preliminary safety and efficacy results of laser immunotherapy for the treatment of metastatic breast cancer patients. Photochem Photobiol Sci. 2011 May;10(5):817-21. PMID: 21373701.	Article did not address use of imaging for treatment evaluation for metastatic breast cancer.
77	Liljegren A, Bergh J, Castany R. Early experience with sunitinib, combined with docetaxel, in patients with metastatic breast cancer. Breast. 2009 Aug;18(4):259-62. PMID: 19744626.	Article did not address use of imaging for treatment evaluation for metastatic breast cancer.
78	Lindholm P, Lapela M, Nagren K, et al. Preliminary study of carbon-11 methionine PET in the evaluation of early response to therapy in advanced breast cancer. Nucl Med Commun. 2009 Jan;30(1):30-6. PMID: 19306512.	Although article published in 2009, PET scans done 1990-1994 using tracer MET, which is now obsolete.
79	Littrup PJ, Jallad B, Chandiwala-Mody P, et al. Cryotherapy for breast cancer: a feasibility study without excision. J Vasc Interv Radiol. 2009 Oct;20(10):1329-41. PMID: 19800542.	Article did not address use of imaging for treatment evaluation for metastatic breast cancer.
80	Lu CY, Srasuebkul P, Drew AK, et al. Positive spillover effects of prescribing requirements: increased cardiac testing in patients treated with trastuzumab for HER2+ metastatic breast cancer. Intern Med J. 2012 Nov;42(11):1229-35. PMID: 21981464.	Article did not address use of imaging for treatment evaluation for metastatic breast cancer.
81	MacDonald SM, Harisinghani MG, Katkar A, et al. Nanoparticle-enhanced MRI to evaluate radiation delivery to the regional lymphatics for patients with breast cancer. Int J Radiat Oncol Biol Phys. 2010 Jul 15;77(4):1098-104. PMID: 19836160.	Article did not address use of imaging for treatment evaluation for metastatic breast cancer.
82	Macia Escalante S, Rodriguez Lescure A, Pons Sanz V, et al. A patient with breast cancer with hepatic metastases and a complete response to herceptin as monotherapy. Clin Transl Oncol. 2006 Oct;8(10):761-3. PMID: 17074677.	Article did not address use of imaging for treatment evaluation for metastatic breast cancer.
83	Maffioli L, Florimonte L, Pagani L, et al. Current role of bone scan with phosphonates in the follow-up of breast cancer. Eur J Nucl Med Mol Imaging. 2004 Jun;31 Suppl 1:S143-8. PMID: 15088128.	Article did not address use of imaging for treatment evaluation for metastatic breast cancer.
84	Malmstrom P, Holmberg L, Anderson H, et al. Breast conservation surgery, with and without radiotherapy, in women with lymph node-negative breast cancer: a randomised clinical trial in a population with access to public mammography screening. Eur J Cancer. 2003 Aug;39(12):1690-7. PMID: 12888363.	Article did not address use of imaging for treatment evaluation for metastatic breast cancer.
85	Mariani G, Erba P, Villa G, et al. Lymphoscintigraphic and intraoperative detection of the sentinel lymph node in breast cancer patients: the nuclear medicine perspective. J Surg Oncol. 2004 Mar;85(3):112-22. PMID: 14991882.	Article did not address use of imaging for treatment evaluation for metastatic breast cancer.
86	Menes TS, Kerlikowske K, Jaffer S, et al. Rates of atypical ductal hyperplasia have declined with less use of postmenopausal hormone treatment: findings from the Breast Cancer Surveillance Consortium. Cancer Epidemiol Biomarkers Prev. 2009 Nov;18(11):2822-8. PMID: 19900937.	Article did not address use of imaging for treatment evaluation for metastatic breast cancer.

Number	Citation	Reason for Exclusion
87	Moadel RM, Nguyen AV, Lin EY, et al. Positron emission tomography agent 2-deoxy-2-[18F]fluoro-D-glucose has a therapeutic potential in breast cancer. Breast Cancer Res. 2003;5(6):R199-205. PMID: 14580255.	Article did not address use of imaging for treatment evaluation for metastatic breast cancer.
88	Montemurro F, Russo F, Martincich L, et al. Dynamic contrast enhanced magnetic resonance imaging in monitoring bone metastases in breast cancer patients receiving bisphosphonates and endocrine therapy. Acta Radiol. 2004 Feb;45(1):71-4. PMID: 15164782.	Article did not address use of imaging for treatment evaluation for metastatic breast cancer.
89	Montgomery DA, Krupa K, Cooke TG. Follow-up in breast cancer: does routine clinical examination improve outcome? A systematic review of the literature. Br J Cancer. 2007 Dec 17;97(12):1632-41. PMID: 18000508.	Article did not address use of imaging for treatment evaluation for metastatic breast cancer.
90	Moon HJ, Kim MJ, Kim EK, et al. US surveillance of regional lymph node recurrence after breast cancer surgery. Radiology. 2009 Sep;252(3):673-81. PMID: 19546429.	Article about imaging to monitor cancer recurrence, not treatment evaluation.
91	Moss S, Waller M, Anderson TJ, et al. Randomised controlled trial of mammographic screening in women from age 40: predicted mortality based on surrogate outcome measures. Br J Cancer. 2005 Mar 14;92(5):955-60. PMID: 15726103.	Article did not address use of imaging for treatment evaluation for metastatic breast cancer.
92	Nagashima T, Sakakibara M, Kadowaki M, et al. Response rate to neoadjuvant chemotherapy measured on imaging predicts early recurrence and death in breast cancer patients with lymph node involvements. Acta Radiol. 2011 Apr 1;52(3):241-6. PMID: 21498357.	Article did not include metastatic breast cancer patients.
93	Nakamura H, Kawasaki N, Taguchi M, et al. Reconstruction of the anterior chest wall after subtotal sternectomy for metastatic breast cancer: report of a case. Surg Today. 2007;37(12):1083-6. PMID: 18030570.	Article did not address use of imaging for treatment evaluation for metastatic breast cancer.
94	Newman LA. Local control of ductal carcinoma in situ based on tumor and patient characteristics: the surgeon's perspective. J Natl Cancer Inst Monogr. 2010;2010(41):152-7. PMID: 20956822.	Article did not address use of imaging for treatment evaluation for metastatic breast cancer.
95	Newstead GM. MR imaging in the management of patients with breast cancer. Semin Ultrasound CT MR. 2006 Aug;27(4):320-32. PMID: 16916000.	Article did not address use of imaging for treatment evaluation for metastatic breast cancer.
96	Newton-Northup JR, Dickerson MT, Ma L, et al. Inhibition of metastatic tumor formation in vivo by a bacteriophage display-derived galectin-3 targeting peptide. Clin Exp Metastasis. 2013 Feb;30(2):119-32. PMID: 22851004.	Article did not address use of imaging for treatment evaluation for metastatic breast cancer.
97	Ngo C, Pollet AG, Laperrelle J, et al. Intraoperative ultrasound localization of nonpalpable breast cancers. Ann Surg Oncol. 2007 Sep;14(9):2485-9. PMID: 17541694.	Article did not address use of imaging for treatment evaluation for metastatic breast cancer.
98	Nirmala S, Krishnaswamy M, Janaki MG, et al. Unilateral solitary choroid metastasis from breast cancer: rewarding results of external radiotherapy. J Cancer Res Ther. 2008 Oct-Dec;4(4):206-8. PMID: 19052398.	Article did not address use of imaging for treatment evaluation for metastatic breast cancer.
99	Ono M, Ando M, Yunokawa M, et al. Brain metastases in patients who receive trastuzumab-containing chemotherapy for HER2-overexpressing metastatic breast cancer. Int J Clin Oncol. 2009 Feb;14(1):48-52. PMID: 19225924.	Article did not address use of imaging for treatment evaluation for metastatic breast cancer.
100	Orgera G, Curigliano G, Krokidis M, et al. High-intensity focused ultrasound effect in breast cancer nodal metastasis. Cardiovasc Intervent Radiol. 2010 Apr;33(2):447-9. PMID: 20162283.	Article did not address use of imaging for treatment evaluation for metastatic breast cancer.
101	Park SH, Kim MJ, Park BW, et al. Impact of preoperative ultrasonography and fine-needle aspiration of axillary lymph nodes on surgical management of primary breast cancer. Ann Surg Oncol. 2011 Mar;18(3):738-44. PMID: 20890729.	Article about diagnostic breast imaging, not imaging for treatment evaluation.

Number	Citation	Reason for Exclusion
102	Pass H, Vicini FA, Kestin LL, et al. Changes in management techniques and patterns of disease recurrence over time in patients with breast carcinoma treated with breast-conserving therapy at a single institution. Cancer. 2004 Aug 15;101(4):713-20. PMID: 15305400.	Article did not address use of imaging for treatment evaluation for metastatic breast cancer.
103	Pavic D, Koomen MA, Kuzmiak CM, et al. The role of magnetic resonance imaging in diagnosis and management of breast cancer. Technol Cancer Res Treat. 2004 Dec;3(6):527-41. PMID: 15560710.	Article did not address use of imaging for treatment evaluation for metastatic breast cancer.
104	Port ER, Yeung H, Gonen M, et al. 18F-2-fluoro-2-deoxy-D-glucose positron emission tomography scanning affects surgical management in selected patients with high-risk, operable breast carcinoma. Ann Surg Oncol. 2006 May;13(5):677-84. PMID: 16538409.	Article did not address use of imaging for treatment evaluation for metastatic breast cancer.
105	Pusztai L, Wagner P, Ibrahim N, et al. Phase II study of tariquidar, a selective P-glycoprotein inhibitor, in patients with chemotherapy-resistant, advanced breast carcinoma. Cancer. 2005 Aug 15;104(4):682-91. PMID: 15986399.	Article did not address use of imaging for treatment evaluation for metastatic breast cancer.
106	Qamri Z, Preet A, Nasser MW, et al. Synthetic cannabinoid receptor agonists inhibit tumor growth and metastasis of breast cancer. Mol Cancer Ther. 2009 Nov;8(11):3117-29. PMID: 19887554.	Article did not address use of imaging for treatment evaluation for metastatic breast cancer.
107	Rades D, Douglas S, Veninga T, et al. Prognostic factors in a series of 504 breast cancer patients with metastatic spinal cord compression. Strahlenther Onkol. 2012 Apr;188(4):340-5. PMID: 22354333.	Article did not address use of imaging for treatment evaluation for metastatic breast cancer.
108	Rebollo-Aguirre AC, Gallego-Peinado M, Menjon-Beltran S, et al. Sentinel lymph node biopsy in patients with operable breast cancer treated with neoadjuvant chemotherapy. Rev Esp Med Nucl Imagen Mol. 2012 May-Jun;31(3):117-23. PMID: 21676504.	Article did not include metastatic breast cancer patients.
109	Rimner A, Rosenzweig KE. Palliative radiation for lung cancer metastases to the breast: two case reports. J Thorac Oncol. 2007 Dec;2(12):1133-5. PMID: 18090590.	Article did not address use of imaging for treatment evaluation for metastatic breast cancer.
110	Roddiger SJ, Kolotas C, Filipowicz I, et al. Neoadjuvant interstitial high-dose-rate (HDR) brachytherapy combined with systemic chemotherapy in patients with breast cancer. Strahlenther Onkol. 2006 Jan;182(1):22-9. PMID: 16404517.	Article did not address use of imaging for treatment evaluation for metastatic breast cancer.
111	Roos DE, Brophy BP, Taylor J. Lessons from a 17-year radiosurgery experience at the Royal Adelaide Hospital. Int J Radiat Oncol Biol Phys. 2012 Jan 1;82(1):102-6. PMID: 21036488.	Article did not address use of imaging for treatment evaluation for metastatic breast cancer.
112	Rousseau C, Devillers A, Campone M, et al. FDG PET evaluation of early axillary lymph node response to neoadjuvant chemotherapy in stage II and III breast cancer patients. Eur J Nucl Med Mol Imaging. 2011 Jun;38(6):1029-36. PMID: 21308372.	Article did not include metastatic breast cancer patients.
113	Ruhl R, Ludemann L, Czarnecka A, et al. Radiobiological restrictions and tolerance doses of repeated single-fraction hdr-irradiation of intersecting small liver volumes for recurrent hepatic metastases. Radiat Oncol. 2010;5:44. PMID: 20507615.	Article did not address use of imaging for treatment evaluation for metastatic breast cancer.
114	Ruhstaller T, von Moos R, Rufibach K, et al. Breast cancer patients on endocrine therapy reveal more symptoms when self-reporting than in pivotal trials: an outcome research study. Oncology. 2009;76(2):142-8. PMID: 19158446.	Article did not address use of imaging for treatment evaluation for metastatic breast cancer.
115	Saito AI, Lightsey J, Li JG, et al. Accuracy of breast cancer axillary lymph node treatment plans based on 2-dimensional imaging: what we should know before interpreting 2-dimensional treatment-planning era studies. Am J Clin Oncol. 2009 Aug;32(4):387-95. PMID: 19546802.	Article did not address use of imaging for treatment evaluation for metastatic breast cancer.
116	Salloum RG, Hornbrook MC, Fishman PA, et al. Adherence to surveillance care guidelines after breast and colorectal cancer treatment with curative intent. Cancer. 2012 Nov 15;118(22):5644-51. PMID: 22434568.	Article did not address use of imaging for treatment evaluation for metastatic breast cancer.

Number	Citation	Reason for Exclusion
117	Sato K, Shigenaga R, Ueda S, et al. Sentinel lymph node biopsy for breast cancer. J Surg Oncol. 2007 Sep 15;96(4):322-9. PMID: 17879334.	Article did not address use of imaging for treatment evaluation for metastatic breast cancer.
118	Seemann MD. Diagnostic value of PET/CT for predicting of neoadjuvant chemotherapy response. Eur J Med Res. 2007 Feb 26;12(2):90-1. PMID: 17369123.	Article did not address use of imaging for treatment evaluation for metastatic breast cancer.
119	Servais EL, Colovos C, Kachala SS, et al. Pre-clinical mouse models of primary and metastatic pleural cancers of the lung and breast and the use of bioluminescent imaging to monitor pleural tumor burden. Curr Protoc Pharmacol. 2011 Sep;Chapter 14:Unit14.21. PMID: 21898334.	Non-human study.
120	Sethi RA, No HS, Jozsef G, et al. Comparison of three-dimensional versus intensity-modulated radiotherapy techniques to treat breast and axillary level III and supraclavicular nodes in a prone versus supine position. Radiother Oncol. 2012 Jan;102(1):74-81. PMID: 21993404.	Article did not address use of imaging for treatment evaluation for metastatic breast cancer.
121	Souchon R, Wenz F, Sedlmayer F, et al. DEGRO practice guidelines for palliative radiotherapy of metastatic breast cancer: bone metastases and metastatic spinal cord compression (MSCC). Strahlenther Onkol. 2009 Jul;185(7):417-24. PMID: 19714302.	Article did not address use of imaging for treatment evaluation for metastatic breast cancer.
122	Spear SL, Clemens MW, Dayan JH. Considerations of previous augmentation in subsequent breast reconstruction. Aesthet Surg J. 2008 May-Jun;28(3):285-93. PMID: 19083539.	Article did not address use of imaging for treatment evaluation for metastatic breast cancer.
123	Sperber F, Weinstein Y, Sarid D, et al. Preoperative clinical, mammographic and sonographic assessment of neoadjuvant chemotherapy response in breast cancer. Isr Med Assoc J. 2006 May;8(5):342-6. PMID: 16805235.	Article did not address use of imaging for treatment evaluation for metastatic breast cancer.
124	Stranzl H, Zurl B, Langsenlehner T, et al. Wide tangential fields including the internal mammary lymph nodes in patients with left-sided breast cancer. Influence of respiratory-controlled radiotherapy (4D-CT) on cardiac exposure. Strahlenther Onkol. 2009 Mar;185(3):155-60. PMID: 19330291.	Article did not address use of imaging for treatment evaluation for metastatic breast cancer.
125	Straver ME, Loo CE, Alderliesten T, et al. Marking the axilla with radioactive iodine seeds (MARI procedure) may reduce the need for axillary dissection after neoadjuvant chemotherapy for breast cancer. Br J Surg. 2010 Aug;97(8):1226-31. PMID: 20602508.	Article did not address use of imaging for treatment evaluation for metastatic breast cancer.
126	Sun G, Jin P, Li M, et al. Percutaneous vertebroplasty for treatment of osteolytic metastases of the C2 vertebral body using anterolateral and posterolateral approach. Technol Cancer Res Treat. 2010 Aug;9(4):417-22. PMID: 20626207.	Article did not address use of imaging for treatment evaluation for metastatic breast cancer.
127	Tisman G. Inhibition of HER2/estrogen receptor cross-talk, probable relation to prolonged remission of stage IV breast cancer: a case report. Tumori. 2009 Nov-Dec;95(6):804-7. PMID: 20210247.	Article did not address use of imaging for treatment evaluation for metastatic breast cancer.
128	Tolentino PJ. Brain metastases secondary to breast cancer: treatment with surgical resection and stereotactic radiosurgery. Mo Med. 2009 Nov-Dec;106(6):428-31. PMID: 20063515.	Article did not address use of imaging for treatment evaluation for metastatic breast cancer.
129	Tomasevic ZI, Rakocevic Z, Tomasevic ZM, et al. Incidence of brain metastases in early stage HER2 3+ breast cancer patients; is there a role for brain CT in asymptomatic patients? J buon. 2012 Apr-Jun;17(2):249-53. PMID: 22740201.	Article addressed diagnosing brain metastases, not evaluating treatment of metastatic breast cancer
130	Trumm CG, Jakobs TF, Zech CJ, et al. CT fluoroscopy-guided percutaneous vertebroplasty for the treatment of osteolytic breast cancer metastases: results in 62 sessions with 86 vertebrae treated. J Vasc Interv Radiol. 2008 Nov;19(11):1596-606. PMID: 18954766.	Article did not address use of imaging for treatment evaluation for metastatic breast cancer.

Number	Citation	Reason for Exclusion
131	Tsai SH, Chen CY, Ku CH, et al. The semiquantitative bone scintigraphy index correlates with serum tartrate-resistant acid phosphatase activity in breast cancer patients with bone metastasis. Mayo Clin Proc. 2007 Aug;82(8):917-26. PMID: 17673059.	Article did not address use of imaging for treatment evaluation for metastatic breast cancer.
132	Wallace AM, Comstock C, Hoh CK, et al. Breast imaging: a surgeon's prospective. Nucl Med Biol. 2005 Oct;32(7):781-92. PMID: 16243654.	Article did not address use of imaging for treatment evaluation for metastatic breast cancer.
133	Wang X, Zhang W, Xu Z, et al. Sonodynamic and photodynamic therapy in advanced breast carcinoma: a report of 3 cases. Integr Cancer Ther. 2009 Sep;8(3):283-7. PMID: 19815599.	Article did not address use of imaging for treatment evaluation for metastatic breast cancer.
134	Wang X, Zhao Y, Cao X. Clinical benefits of mastectomy on treatment of occult breast carcinoma presenting axillary metastases. Breast J. 2010 Jan-Feb;16(1):32-7. PMID: 20465598.	Article did not address use of imaging for treatment evaluation for metastatic breast cancer.
135	Wieners G, Mohnike K, Peters N, et al. Treatment of hepatic metastases of breast cancer with CT-guided interstitial brachytherapy - a phase II-study. Radiother Oncol. 2011 Aug;100(2):314-9. PMID: 21497930.	Article did not address use of imaging for treatment evaluation for metastatic breast cancer.
136	Wiggenraad R, Verbeek-de Kanter A, Mast M, et al. Local progression and pseudo progression after single fraction or fractionated stereotactic radiotherapy for large brain metastases. A single centre study. Strahlenther Onkol. 2012 Aug;188(8):696-701. PMID: 22722818.	Article did not address use of imaging for treatment evaluation for metastatic breast cancer.
137	Wilbert J, Guckenberger M, Polat B, et al. Semi-robotic 6 degree of freedom positioning for intracranial high precision radiotherapy; first phantom and clinical results. Radiat Oncol. 2010;5:42. PMID: 20504338.	Article did not address use of imaging for treatment evaluation for metastatic breast cancer.
138	Wiseman CL, Kharazi A. Objective clinical regression of metastatic breast cancer in disparate sites after use of whole-cell vaccine genetically modified to release sargramostim. Breast J. 2006 Sep-Oct;12(5):475-80. PMID: 16958969.	Article did not address use of imaging for treatment evaluation for metastatic breast cancer.
139	Yasojima H, Shimomura A, Naoi Y, et al. Association between c-myc amplification and pathological complete response to neoadjuvant chemotherapy in breast cancer. Eur J Cancer. 2011 Aug;47(12):1779-88. PMID: 21741827.	Article did not include metastatic breast cancer patients.
140	Yavetz D, Corn BW, Matceyevsky D, et al. Improved treatment of the breast and supraclavicular fossa based on a simple geometrical principle. Med Dosim. 2011 Winter;36(4):434-9. PMID: 21397491.	Article did not address use of imaging for treatment evaluation for metastatic breast cancer.
141	Yen CP, Sheehan J, Patterson G, et al. Gamma knife surgery for metastatic brainstem tumors. J Neurosurg. 2006 Aug;105(2):213-9. PMID: 17219825.	Article did not address use of imaging for treatment evaluation for metastatic breast cancer.
142	Yu JC, Hsu GC, Hsieh CB, et al. Role of sentinel lymphadenectomy combined with intraoperative ultrasound in the assessment of locally advanced breast cancer after neoadjuvant chemotherapy. Ann Surg Oncol. 2007 Jan;14(1):174-80. PMID: 17066228.	Article did not include metastatic breast cancer patients.

Appendix E. Literature Flow Diagram

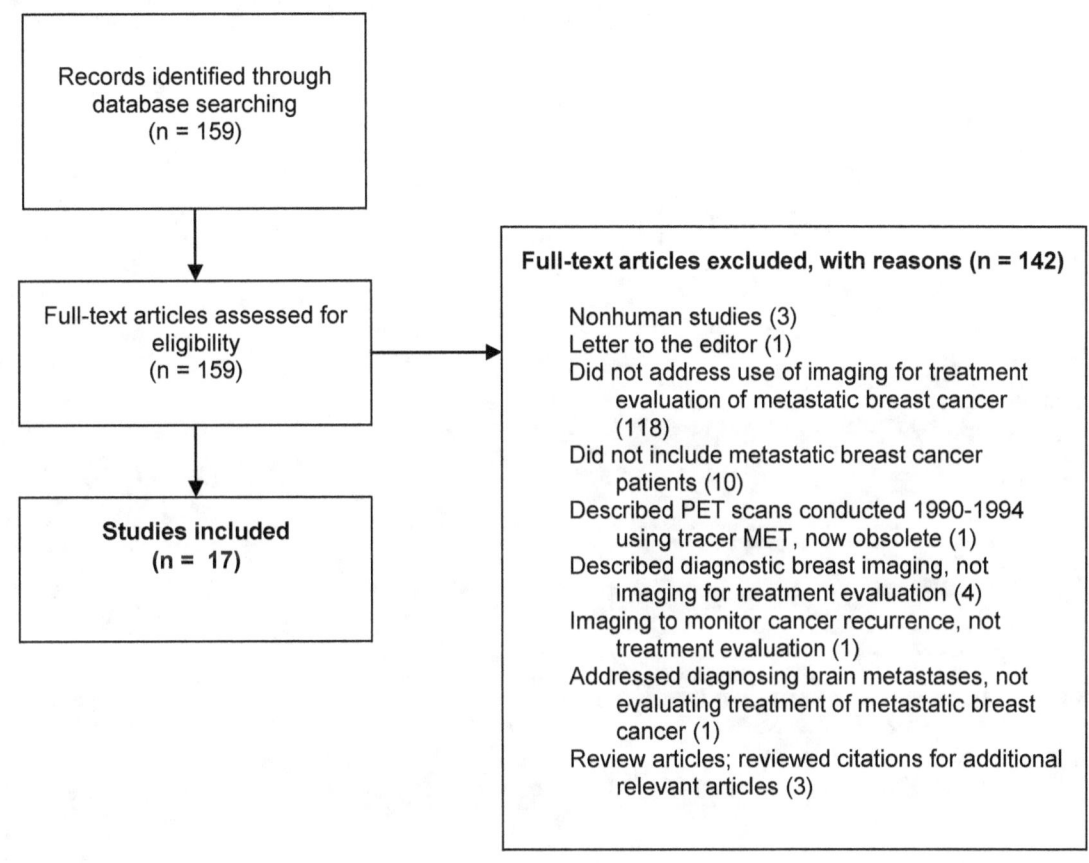

Records identified through
database searching
(n = 159)

Full-text articles assessed for
eligibility
(n = 159)

Studies included
(n = 17)

Full-text articles excluded, with reasons (n = 142)

Nonhuman studies (3)
Letter to the editor (1)
Did not address use of imaging for treatment
evaluation of metastatic breast cancer
(118)
Did not include metastatic breast cancer
patients (10)
Described PET scans conducted 1990-1994
using tracer MET, now obsolete (1)
Described diagnostic breast imaging, not
imaging for treatment evaluation (4)
Imaging to monitor cancer recurrence, not
treatment evaluation (1)
Addressed diagnosing brain metastases, not
evaluating treatment of metastatic breast
cancer (1)
Review articles; reviewed citations for additional
relevant articles (3)

Appendix F. Calculation of Estimate of Number of Women Receiving Imaging for Treatment Evaluation of Metastatic Breast Cancer

We estimated that the U.S. prevalence of women with metastatic breast cancer is about 160,000, with a median survival time of about 2 years.[1] Our Key Informants estimated that about 90 percent of women with metastatic breast cancer receive some type of chemotherapy and that treatment for metastatic breast cancer typically lasts about 1 year. We estimated that about half of the 160,000 women, or about 80,000 women, would be in the first year of their metastatic breast cancer diagnosis and would be candidates for receiving treatment, and 90 percent of these, or 72,000, would be receiving chemotherapy and thus imaging for treatment evaluations per year. Our literature search covered 11 years, so 72,000*11=792,000 women received scans for treatment evaluation of metastatic breast cancer.

---

[1] Metastatic Breast Cancer Network. Education: Prevalence of Metastatic Breast Cancer. 2013. http://mbcn.org/education/category/prevalence/. Accessed on December 16, 2013.

www.ingramcontent.com/pod-product-compliance
Lightning Source LLC
Chambersburg PA
CBHW081741170526
45167CB00009B/3899